CBD Oil: The #1 Ultimate Beginners Guide

By

Les Brown

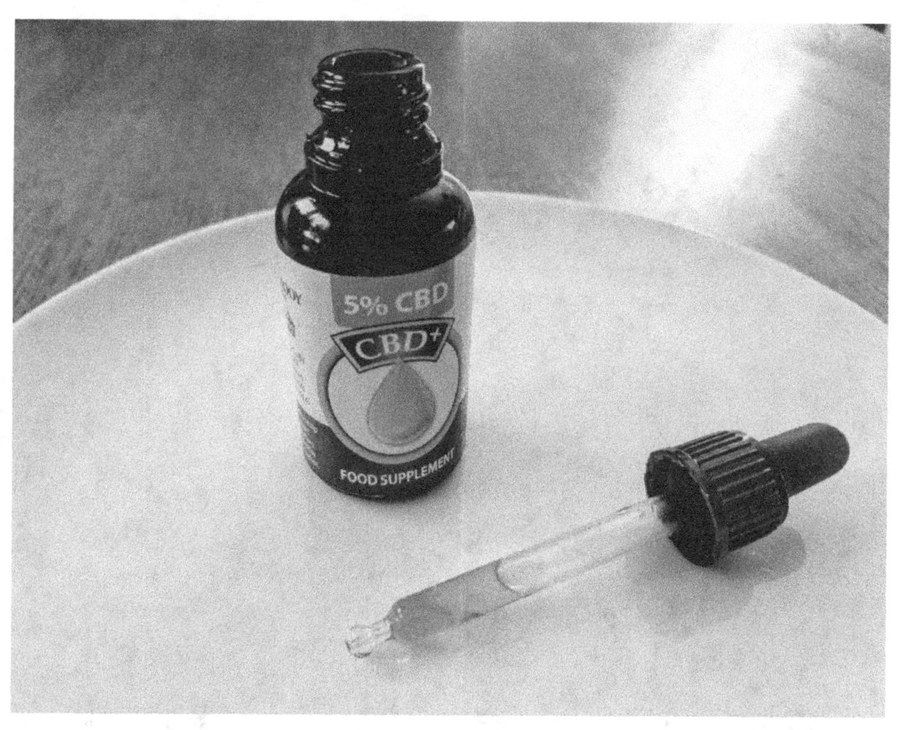

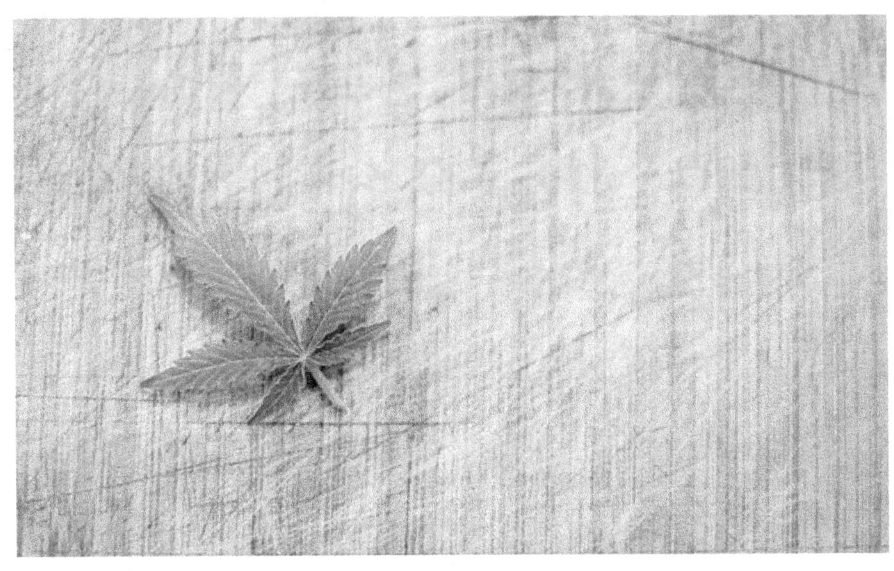

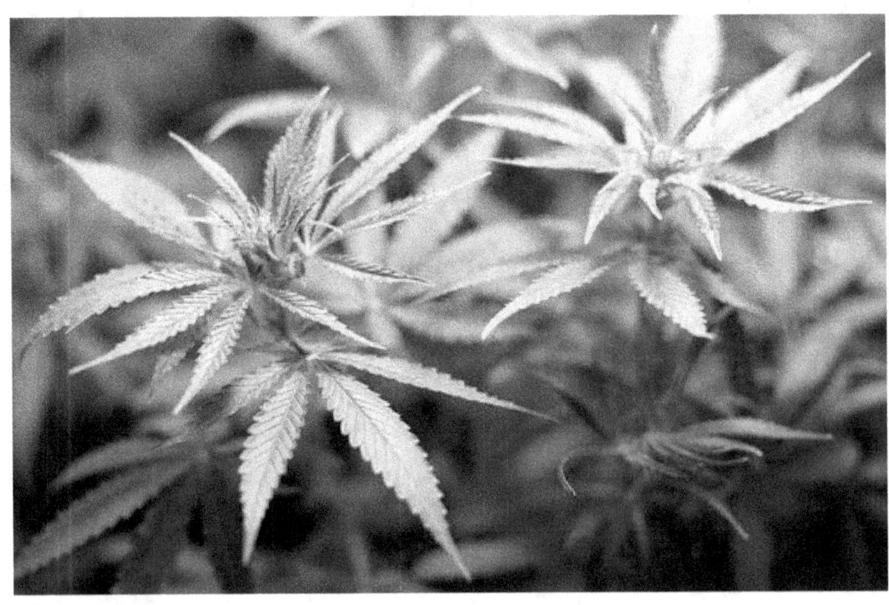

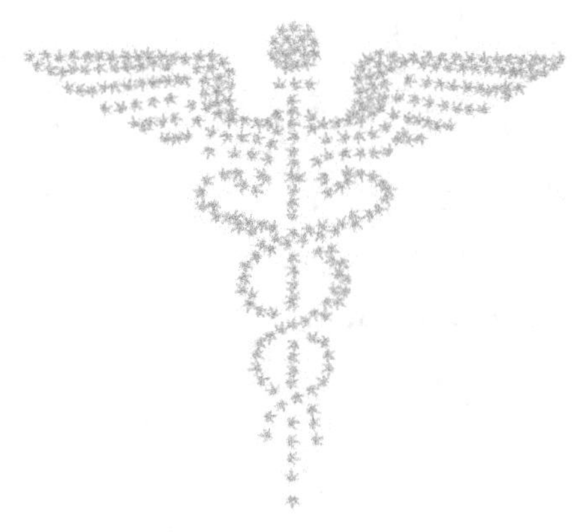

Contents

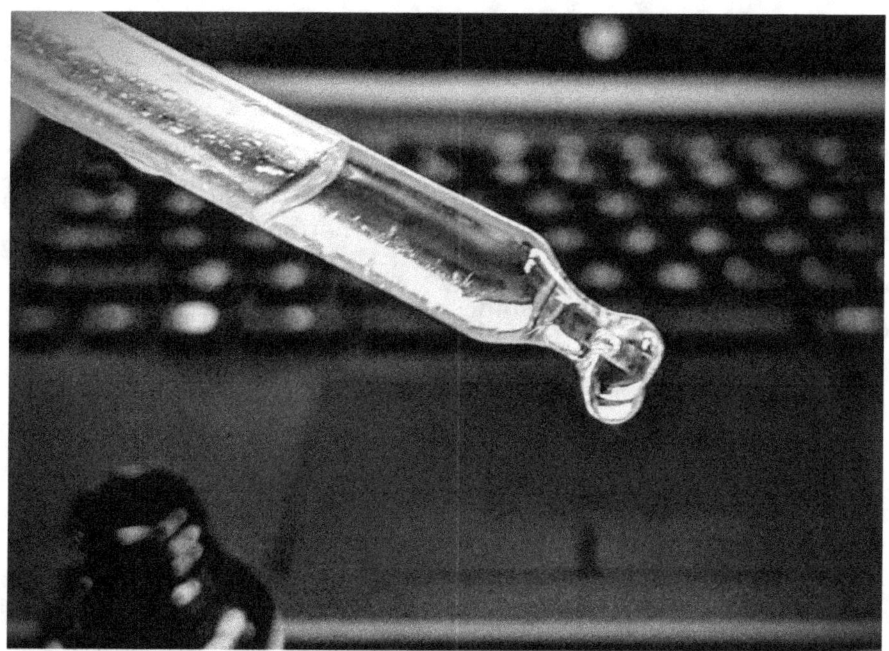

The following eBook is reproduced with the goal of providing information that is as accurate and reliable as possible. The recommendations suggestions contained in these pages are solely for entertainment purposes. Before undertaking any action based on the contents of this book, consult a medical health professional.

This declaration is deemed fair and valid by both the American Bar Association and the Committee of Publishers Association and is legally binding throughout the United States.

Furthermore, the transmission duplication or reproduction of any of the following work in any form (including specific information) is illegal. This extends to creating a secondary or tertiary copy of the work. No record copy of this work can me produced without with the express, written consent from the publisher. All additional rights reserved.

The information in the following pages is broadly considered to be a truthful and accurate account of facts and, as such, any inattention, use or misuse of the information in question by the reader will render any resulting actions solely under his/her purview. There are no instances in which the publisher or the original author of this work can be deemed liable for any hardship or damages that may befall them after undertaking information described herein.

Additionally, the information in the following pages is intended only for informational purposes and should thus be regarded as universal. As befitting its nature, it is presented without assurance regarding its prolonged validity or interim quality. Trademarks that are mentioned are done without written consent and can in no way be considered an endorsement from the trademark holder.

This book in no way endorses or glamourizes any type of criminal or illegal activity including any type of illegal consumption of drugs, or anything linked to illegal drugs, drug paraphernalia, beating drug tests or any claims of medical uses whatsoever.

Preface

Congratulations and thank you for buying this book. I am thrilled to have the opportunity to share my knowledge and experience with you and I really do hope that you enjoy reading it as much as I enjoyed writing it for you.

You have almost certainly already heard about the miraculous healing powers of CBD oil or perhaps you've read about it on the internet, or in a magazine or through your social media news feeds, and it has piqued your interest. A quick Google search will probably have thrown up lots of conflicting information about the health benefits along with what is in CBD oil and whether it's legal.

The truth is that CBD is a fascinating and often confusing subject to get to grips with. There is currently a lack of Scientific data available on the apparent health benefits and the laws that surround CBD in some countries are mixed and varied. Even buying CBD oil is a bit of a minefield.

Understanding exactly what CBD can is be confusing given the number of inconsistent facts that you'll find in other books or online. I have found that buying and using the right CBD oil for your personal circumstances can get a bit overwhelming unless you know what you're doing.

To add to this, when I first started researching CBD oil to help treat my parents ailments, it struck me that most of the books I read were either written by people who had never actually taken the oil themselves, or by people who owned or had an affiliate relationship with a Hemp related company and who were selling CBD Hemp products.

Now there is nothing at all wrong with that of course however let's be honest here. Would you for example, prefer to take advice about a second-hand car from the used car salesman who's trying to sell it to you or would you rather listen to a previous owner who knew the car inside and out and had no interest in whether you buy the car? I know which one is more likely to give you the facts that you need to know. It's the same when it comes to learning about CBD oil.

Being a practicing Herbalist and Nutritionist I wanted to cut through all the hype and sales chat and get to the kind of real, unbiased and unfiltered insight that only learned knowledge coupled with applied personal experience can provide.

It was during my intense research that I decided that the best way for me to experience what it was really like to search, buy, use and live with a suitable type of CBD oil was to roll up my sleeves and to go through the process for myself. This first-hand experience would provide the real answers to my questions.

What I discovered was pretty eye opening and unexpected. Lots of so-called CBD products for sale didn't contain any CBD in them at all and the nutritional value and alleged benefits were often questionable at best. Some items are labelled in such a way which can make it easy for consumers to waste time and money on products which will simply not work for them.

I was quite shocked when I discovered that the current upturn in the CBD market has led to some unscrupulous sellers to try to take advantage of people's inexperience of this product and they are in turn being economical with the truth in describing their products merits to cash in on a booming trade.

Over time my inquisitive and curious nature has led me to experiment with various brands, strengths, methods of consumption and dosage to find what really works best for me. I have often pushed the boundaries at times to discover facts about CBD oil which were not available either in books or online.

It has been extremely rewarding for me to be able to help lead many clients along with my family and (furry) friends towards a pain free life and to help them feel less anxious, fitter and more energized. I've witnessed some amazing transformations in people and animals and it's really exciting for me to be able to be able to share my experience with you and to help you finally become free from pain and anxiety.

This book contains everything that you should know about getting started with CBD oil. In it you will gain the benefit of my own personal research and practical experience as a buyer and user of CBD oil to treat my own ailments and to help me with my health and fitness goals.

I will guide you step by step and take you from complete beginner level to a CBD Black Belt in under two hours. You will then be able to confidently apply this knowledge and lead a fuller, happier life.

Thanks again for buying this book. I really hope that you enjoy it.

Are you ready?

Now let's get started!

Introduction

When you hear the word cannabis what's the first thought that pops into your head?

Hippies? Bob Marley? Student Politicians who allegedly didn't inhale?

Whatever you thought it probably included someone engulfed in a cloud of smoke as they puff on a large joint.

That's because to most people cannabis is illegal marijuana, and marijuana gets people high. The thing is, what most people don't realize is that there is more to it than that. A lot more.

Cannabis plants contain over 100 chemical compounds called cannabinoids. Two of the main cannabinoids are THC (tetrahydrocannabinol) and CBD (cannabidiol)

Okay now let's get something nice and sparkly clear before we move on.

THC gets you high whereas CBD doesn't.

Cannabis plants come in different species including Marijuana and Industrial Hemp. Both marijuana and hemp fall under the generic umbrella term cannabis however they are both very different.

Hemp comes from the cannabis sativa plant and marijuana comes from the cannabis Indica variety.

Cannabis sativa plants were found in Europe and Western Eurasia, where it was cultivated for its fiber and seeds.

On the other hand, Cannabis Indica encompasses the psychoactive varieties found in India where it was harvested for its fiber, seeds and production of hashish.

Marijuana comes from the Cannabis Indica variety and is still illegal in most countries as it contains high levels of THC which as we've said, can get you high.

Hemp however is perfectly legal in most countries as it contains mostly CBD with trace amounts of THC. Hemp therefore will not get you high.

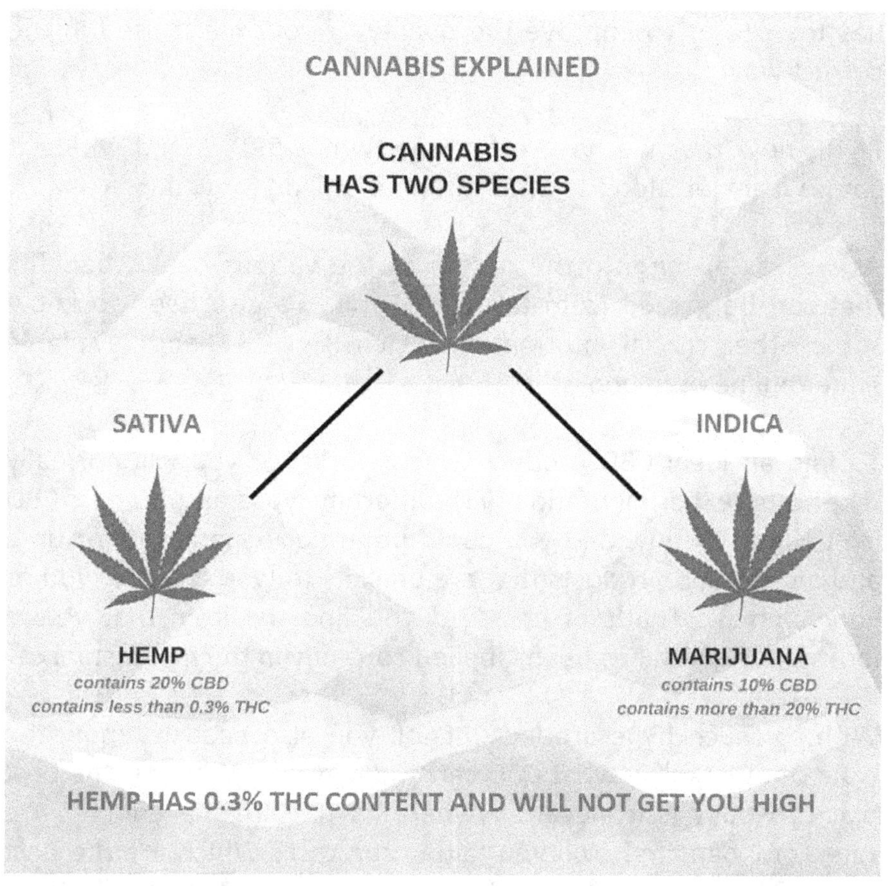

Despite the current surge in popularity, cannabis isn't new. It's one of our oldest crops and we have used it in some form or other for thousands of years.

The Chinese Emperor Shen Nung used it in 2727 BC. Ancient Greeks, Romans and Egyptians used it as did the Vikings and just about every other race and culture that you can think of including the Royal Family. Why? Because it is a robust and extremely versatile plant that we can utilize to benefit us in literally thousands of ways. It's extremely valuable to us and put simply it has the power to improve the quality of your life if used in the correct way.

Right, now that we have established what CBD is and where it comes from let's look at what this book will do for you.

As well as diving into the details of the various health benefits that can be gained from taking CBD oil, we also need to know some other crucial information which isn't as readily available either online or in books.

To find an ideal CBD product which works for you will normally take some experimentation with different types and brands. CBD isn't cheap to buy, and you could potentially spend lots of time and money and products that are unlikely to work best for you or your animals. That's of course if you find the item that you're looking for which has been labelled correctly in the first instance.

With so much hype around CBD oil you also need to know the truth about exactly what CBD can and can't do. Where is the best place to buy? Is it illegal anywhere? What are the effects? Are there any dangers? Will you fail a drug test? Which are the best brands? Can you mix brands? Can you mix with other medications or alcohol? How much can you expect to spend? The best methods of consumption? How to read the often-confusing labels?

This book has been written to give you concise knowledge on all aspects of CBD and to save you time and money.

It has been written in easy to understand terms with the facts summarized by bullet points for quick and easy access. I really do hope that you love it and that it changes your life.

If you do feel happy with what you have learned from this book, then please take two minutes to leave me a review. It's quick and easy to leave a review and it honestly would mean a lot to me. Thank you in advance.

Are you ready to learn what all the fuss is about and to see what CBD can do for you?

I'm ready. Let's do this together.

Chapter 1:

What exactly is CBD and Hemp Oil?

What is CBD Oil?

CBD oil is what you get when you take cannabinoids from the cannabis sativa plant and mix them with a carrier oil, like coconut, rapeseed, olive or hemp seed oil. CBD is usually extracted from the cannabis plant as an oil or a powder. This oil or powder can then be mixed with a gel or cream that can be rubbed onto the skin or ingested orally.

The cannabis plants contain many cannabinoids which work alongside our bodies own endocannabinoid system (ECS) in ways that are still being discovered. Until recently, THC or tetrahydrocannabinol was the most commonly known of these compounds due to its ability to make the user feel high when consumed.

CBD or Cannabidiol (pronounced cann-a-bid-EYE-ol) has been brought into focus more recently as it's been recognized that it is full of antioxidants and doesn't contain the psychoactive properties of THC. In-fact CBD counter acts the effects of THC.

CBD oil is cannabis oil that has a high content of cannabidiol. It is made from the flowers, leaves and stalks of hemp and not from its seeds like hemp seed oil. The CBD oil can then be stored in tinctures or jars where it will remain fresh in a cupboard for a year or 6 months once opened.

CBD is perfectly safe and has been used as a natural remedy for thousands of years. CBD tolerates mild to moderate heat well and can be mixed into most edibles or even smoothies or cocktails.

CBD oil can be used to naturally treat humans and animals for a variety of ailments without the side effects of conventional synthetic medicine. CBD can also be used to make effective natural beauty products and anti-aging lotion. CBD is also big business. The U.S. market alone for CBD products is estimated to be worth $2.1 Billion by 2020, up 700 percent from 2016.

It's little wonder that CBD can make improve your health and make you feel better. Full spectrum CBD oil is nutritionally dense. It contains:

- Protein
- Fiber
- Essential Fatty Acids. Omega 3 and 6
- Vitamins A, C, E, B1, B2, B3, B6
- Iron
- Beta Carotene
- Zinc

- Potassium
- Calcium
- Selenium
- Phosphorous
- Manganese
- Magnesium
- Flavonoids
- Terpenes
- Terpenoids

CBD oil uses:

- Help manage symptoms of various mental and physical conditions including:
- Insomnia
- Anxiety
- Addiction
- Anti-inflammatory
- Helps treat animals for arthritis and joint pain
- Beauty products
- Health Supplement
- Pain Management

What is Hemp Oil?

Hemp oil or extract must have a THC content of 0.3% or less to be legal in most countries. Hemp oil is extracted by cold pressing the seeds of the hemp plant. Industrial hemp is the only plant used to obtain hemp oil. Hemp oil contains some CBD however in lower amounts than CBD Oil.

Hemp is highly nutritious and extremely versatile and has been used for centuries in the production of textiles, clothing and rope etc. Even today hemp continues to be used in over 26000 products including building materials, moisturizer, paper, plastics, paints and even bio diesel fuel and much more besides. Hemp is still illegal to grow in most countries however possessing hemp oil is not illegal.

Hemp is favored for its wide range of uses whereas CBD oil is more known for its therapeutic qualities. Because of its CBD content hemp oil is packed with nutrients and omega 3 and 6 fatty acids and has been shown to increase memory and concentration. It has also been known to help protect against strokes and heart attacks.

Hemp oil uses:

- Cooking (highly nutritious with a nutty flavor)
- Natural Moisturizer
- Base for different types of plastic
- Eco friendly paint production
- Bio diesel fuel like other vegetable oils
- Making lotions, soaps and foods.
- Hemp Essential Oil.

(Hemp Essential Oil is obtained from the upper leaves and flowers of the hemp plant and is extracted by low-pressure steam distillation. Hemp essential oil offers a wide range of health enhancing benefits including anti-depressant, anti-bacterial and anti-inflammatory affects.)

Points to remember:

- CBD has 0.3% or less THC content and will not get you high.
- Hemp has been used for thousands of years.
- CBD is favored for its potential healing properties.
- Hemp oil is made from the hemp seeds and has a variety of uses.
- Certain sellers of hemp products often have no CBD in them, and the health claims are sometimes being exaggerated.
- CBD and Hemp although different are used in naming CBD Hemp related products like CBD Hemp oil.
- CBD can be produced from combining Hemp seed oil and Hemp paste from the leaves and flowers of the industrial Hemp plant.

Chapter 2:

Our ECS explained

What is the Endocannabinoid System?

The endogenous cannabinoid system was only discovered a few decades ago. The ECS is found in humans and mammals and is an important physiologic system involved in establishing and maintaining our over-all health. Endocannabinoids and their receptors can be found throughout the entire body: in the brain, organs, all connective tissues, glands, and immune cells.

The cannabinoid system performs different tasks; however, the main goal is always for homeostasis within the body. Homeostasis means "the tendency towards a relatively stable equilibrium between interdependent elements, especially as maintained by physiological processes". Balance in other words.

Homeostasis can be challenged by things like air quality, toxins, bad diet and stress etc. When this happens, the body does not naturally produce the right number of endocannabinoids and the ones that are produced are not regulated well enough. The result can be disease, illness, and general poor health.

Endocannabinoids and cannabinoids can also be found in the body's various other systems, allowing for communication and coordination between the different cell types. When a person is injured, cannabinoids will decrease the release of activators and sensitizers from the injured area. They also stabilize the nerve cell to prevent excessive firing, and at the same time calm nearby immune cells to prevent release of pro-inflammatory substances. These actions minimize the pain and damage caused by the injury.

Scientists have found that our clever little ECS is an inter-connected series of mechanisms made of three main components including:

- Cells that allow the receipt and the transmission of cannabinoid receptors.

- Specific enzymes tasked with creating or eliminating cannabinoids; and,

- Endocannabinoids, which the body can produce naturally and will resemble cannabinoid compounds.

These three-parts foster communication inside the body and allow the various biological responses and functions to work well and promote homeostasis. Whenever the balance of the body is compromised, the endocannabinoid system will kick in and try to produce more cannabinoids naturally.

The endocannabinoid system works with:

- Moderating and boosting brain signals
- Enriching connective tissue
- Regulation of organs and glands
- Influence on the immune system
- Mood
- Pain responses
- Energy levels
- Pleasure and the reward centers inside the brain
- Motor control
- Sleep
- Immune function
- Digestion, appetite, and hunger
- Memory
- Regulating body temperature
- Reproduction and fertility

Scientists have given the label of Clinical Endocannabinoid Deficiency Syndrome, or CEDS, to the state when this system is weakened or compromised because the balance is disrupted. Since these molecules are like messengers in the body, any deviation from the norm can result in potential health problems.

When CEDS occurs, the body cannot produce enough of its own cannabinoids. If this happens the individual will lack enough messengers to help regulate their systems, making it challenge to feel fit and healthy and making the person more susceptible to disease and illness.

Supplementing the body with more cannabinoids in the form of CBD oil could help to regulate the body naturally, at least until the body is fit enough to be able to do it independently.

Points to remember:

- The ECS is found in humans and mammals and is vital to your overall health.
- CEDS can occur when the ECS is weakened through biological or external factors
- Cannabinoids promote hemostasis or 'balance' in the body.
- Supplementing with CBD oil could restore balance throughout the body's systems.

Chapter 3:

The Health Benefits of CBD oil.

How CBD oil works

All cannabinoids work by attaching themselves to receptors inside the body to produce their effects. It is natural for the body itself to produce some cannabinoids on its own. The human body has two main receptors for cannabinoids known as the CB1 and CB2 receptors.

The CB1 receptors are found all over the body, which means you could use these cannabinoids pretty much everywhere. However, most of these receptors are found in the brain.

The CB1 receptors in the brain deal with all kinds of movement and coordination along with memories, appetite, thinking, mood and emotions, and even pain. THC attaches specifically to these receptors. Effects can generally take from 20 minutes to up to three hours – the time often depends on the amount consumed and the method of consumption.

On the other hand, the CB2 receptors are more commonly found in the immune system. They work to reduce pain and inflammation in the body.

The thoughts surrounding how CBD oil works have changed recently. It was once believed that CBD acted with the CB2 receptors. However, it now seems that CBD oil does not really react with either receptor in a direct manner. Instead, it works to influence the body to use more of its own natural cannabinoids to get things done.

How long do the effects last?

When you take CBD in any form, it will stay in your system between three to five days. The length of stay depends on the amount you took – and absorption rates vary among people. If you are going to complete a drug test or anything similar, it is important to note that the CBD, even if you just take it only a few times, may possibly register on the test depending on the THC content of your product. Standard drug tests are looking for any THC in your body so technically you should be fine with most CBD oil as 0.3% isn't enough to show a reading on the test. I myself have bought over the counter drug tests and mine showed up perfectly fine even though I have been taking CBD oil with a THC content of 0.2% for a long time.

Even though the CBD can stay in your system for a few days, the effects are only going to last between three to four hours for most people. If you are using CBD to help with common ailments like the ones we have discussed, you may only need to take it a few times a day to keep receiving the benefits. We'll go into dosage more later in the book.

If you are using CBD as a health tonic, then you will know within a few days whether your chosen product is working for you or not. Remember not to expect fireworks initially though. The benefits aren't always immediately obvious, and you should give yourself a few days to a week before trying another brand.

Short-term effects of CBD oil

The short-term effects of CBD oil vary based on who takes it and the condition(s) they have. Some people will report relief from very visible maladies (like seizures). Others simply report a better feeling of general wellness, such as feeling less stress or being able to sleep better. Still others tell of reduced inflammation as CBD works with the body's receptors to relieve pain and to reduce swelling.

The way that you feel will depend on the condition you are treating.

If you are dealing with a more serious condition, you should notice some obvious signs of improvement again within a short time. It depends on a few factors. Sometimes it takes a bit longer to see improvement (based on the type and severity of the condition you face). The good news is that those who take this oil to help with a related health condition report that they feel better even after a relatively short time. I've read that you need to go through a preliminary loading phase before you feel results however not in my experience. I felt the effects and noticed improvements quite quickly. Sometimes even within an hour.

It's important to note that each person will react differently – just as with any other medicine or regimen. I myself have sometimes felt more relaxed and focused shortly after I take my oil when using CBD to relax. Other times I have not felt much different while taking the same dose of the same oil, so I guess your mood and how you're feeling overall that day can have an influence. However, when specifically treating pain like, say a headache then your mood shouldn't play a part in it. The brand of oil that you are using will either work or it won't. As I say each person is unique and will respond differently to different brands and consumption methods.

The golden rule when starting out is always start with a low dosage and see how you feel. As you progress, you can adjust the amount you ingest. Be as objective as possible – it might be advisable to write down your observations and keep a diary for future reference. There doesn't appear to be any real negative short-term effects of taking CBD oil that I have found. I have found no negative short-term effects.

The long-term effects of CBD oil

The long-term effects (like short-term) will again depend on the disorder you are treating, and your individual make up. To date, research has not uncovered any negative, long-term effects for people using the oil to improve their overall health and wellbeing.

If you are suffering from a disorder such as inflammation, headaches, or seizures, you can take this oil as you determine on a regular, daily basis. Whether you decide to use the oil on a regular or occasional basis, CBD is safe and effective to take for the long-term if needed.

I have seen no adverse effects to taking CBD for the long term. It's not addictive. There are no real side effects. I have stopped then started using CBD again and it still has an effect. The only drawback really was the expense of the oil itself. I could easily spend more than $150.00 per month and that doesn't include my expensive product trials and experiments to find what works for me. It's best to get it on prescription of possible where you live. Again, no real negatives to my long-term use. I would however say that occasionally when I suddenly stop using the oil my body and mind sometimes re-adjust and my sleeping pattern is very slightly disturbed for a couple of days. Not a major issue just something that I've noticed. It goes back to normal again with no problems.

Health Benefits of CBD

Specifically, designed CBD oil with a higher THC content of 0.3% has been shown to reduce the size of tumors however generally speaking CBD can be effective at naturally managing the symptoms of various ailments as opposed to curing them at their root cause. CBD is natural and organic and while it can possess minor side effects in some people these are generally very mild compared with some of the quite significant side effects from many of the chemically synthetic conventional medicines which are currently being used to treat the same ailments. CBD has been shown to have a very positive effect upon:

- ADHD
- Acne
- Alzheimer's disease
- Alcoholism
- Anti-biotic resistant infections
- Stroke
- Anxiety Disorders
- Autism
- Type A Diabetes
- Burnout
- Inflammation
- Depression
- Rheumatoid Arthritis
- Eating disorders
- Nicotine addiction
- Dyslexia
- Schizophrenia
- IBS

- Cancer
- Tension
- Seizures
- MS
- Mad Cow Disease
- Epilepsy
- Sleeping disorders
- Crohn's disease
- Hunters disease
- Heart disease
- High Blood pressure
- Chronic Pain
- Opioids
- Headaches
- Pain during childbirth
- Parkinson's
- Psoriasis
- PTSD
- And much more

It can also potentially boost your mental capacity, memory, concentration, athletic endurance and your body's ability to build muscle and burn fat. Quite an impressive list don't you think.

I have personally experienced an increase in my own fitness-levels, and I have managed to build some muscle and lose fat albeit as part of a healthy lifestyle **and** CBD oil. CBD oil has certainly helped me with this however I don't believe that a person could take CBD oil on its own, not exercise and then eat fish and chips for breakfast, lunch and dinner and expect to lose fat. It won't happen.

The same goes for anxiety, depression and insomnia. I believe that CBD should be viewed as a supplement to help or assist with your other efforts to relax more or get fit and not a magic bullet to transform your health and fitness despite living a very unhealthy lifestyle. I expect you'll get more out of CBD oil if you view it this way and wish to use it as a health tonic.

If CBD is intended to be used to treat a health condition like arthritis, epilepsy or cancer then this is quite different. In this instance a person will expect CBD oil to perform the task of reducing pain or the number of fits a patient has and improving the quality of a person's life. The right type of CBD oil should do this. As we discussed earlier there are several cannabinoids other than CBD and THC. Some of these also have benefits and are listed on the chart below.

Let's take a closer look

Many people chose to consider the benefits of CBD oil because they are dealing with health issues and have tried everything else without success. They may have tried all kinds of other treatments and medications, but their symptoms do not diminish – sometimes they even get worse.

CBD can be an effective treatment and often exceeds the performance of traditional medicine. While it may not work for every single person it is worth trying because the risks are minimal and if it works for you it will really change your life for the better.

Cancer and chemotherapy

CBD helps patients deal with the effects of chemotherapy. Those who struggle with, or become sick from, chemotherapy can take CBD oil to help deal with nausea. This could make it a little easier to get through the treatments because you may then have more of an appetite and can eat more and in turn have more energy.

CBD can also help elevate your mood. Patients who are feeling down and understandably upset about their diagnoses may find that CBD helps lift their spirits just a little. Having a positive attitude is of course very important during these very tough times.

 A group of specialists at the National Cancer Institute reviewed experiments with rhesus monkeys and rodents. The results of these studies implied that CBD can inhibit the division of cancerous cells, especially when it came to cancers like lymphoma and leukemia. The CBD chemical was also able to lower the probability that the affected tissue would spread over to other parts of the body. In addition, it can increase the effectiveness of the macrophage cells that attack the cancerous cells in the body.

CBD medications could in time even be used as a replacement treatment to chemotherapy altogether. Some patients have been able to take the CBD medications to stop the cancer by inhibiting the cells from dividing and growing. Since the cells can no longer divide, they begin to die.

CBD also helps prevent the cancerous cells from moving to other parts of the body. When combined with other treatments, it works to keep the cancer localized and can make healing and recovering much easier. CBD with a much higher THC content has been shown to reduce the size of various tumors in some patients. A THC content of up to 90% can be used in this instance.

Heart disease and diabetes

CBD oil carries many anti-inflammatory properties, which we will discuss in more detail later. CBD has been shown to reduce cholesterol levels in the blood. Consequently, it can help with both diabetes and heart disease. First, because of the anti-inflammatory properties, insulin resistance is reduced, which leads to a better prognosis in many patients by lowering the incidence of dead tissue in the body.

Since CBD was discovered in the 1990s, there has been speculation on its effect on other types of receptors in the body, not just on cannabinoid receptors, and whether it could be manipulated and included in various treatment options for cardiovascular diseases like atherosclerosis.

Researchers at the University of Tel Aviv completed studies that showed a 30 percent increase in blood flow in rodents with areas of dead tissue in the heart muscle.

This is positive news for those suffering from either heart disease or diabetes. CBD could reduce your insulin resistance which makes it easier to prevent or manage your diabetes, especially if you do it along with a healthy lifestyle and a healthy diet. Additionally, you can keep your heart healthy and reduce the issues that come with areas of dead tissue leading to the heart. With Heart disease on the increase, you can understand why an increasing number of men and women are looking to try CBD oil. I live in the west of Scotland which is the heart attack capital of the World. This benefit of CBD was of interest to me.

Muscle spasms and seizures

There are many documented cases of children and adults who suffered from extreme seizure disorders, terrible situations where no other treatments had helped, who began to take CBD oil with miraculous results. Their seizures stopped or became very minimal. CBD provided a natural cure, and some claim it has saved their lives.

The FDA currently allows epilepsy centers throughout the United States to prescribe products that contain CBD to patients, if these patients are not responding to classical medication.

A 2015 comprehensive study focusing on Lennox-Gastaut Syndrome and Dravet Syndrome (two very difficult forms of epilepsy) is responsible for the change in treatment protocols. Uncovering the correct treatment and dosage in these two conditions had been very challenging. Children using CBD oil exhibited marked improvement – in some cases, seizures disappeared completely.

Those who took cannabidiol medication for six months found a decrease between 54 and 67 percent. It is important to note that the CBD oil is effective, but it does not work in every patient. There were some participants in the study above who stopped the treatment after three months because it did not improve their conditions at all.

More studies are needed to demonstrate how and why CBD oil works and to determine why is helps some patients but not others. Still, the future looks promising and more research will uncover more potential benefits and pitfalls.

Chronic pain

Looking for effective chronic pain medications is a challenge. Many drugs also have nasty side effects, especially if you take them over the long term. You could even become addicted to these medications.

Now If over-the-counter drugs do not provide relief, your doctor will likely prescribe stronger medications, such as muscle relaxants, anxiety drugs like diazepam/Valium or antidepressants like duloxetine/Cymbalta (musculoskeletal pain), prescription NSAIDs celecoxib/Celebrex or a course of strong painkillers like codeine, fentanyl/Duragesic, Actiq, oxycodone and acetaminophen Percoat, Roxicet, Tylox or sometimes hydrocodone and acetaminophen/Lorcet, Lortab, and Vicodin. You may even require having localized steroid injections to relieve swelling and inflammation. An epidural may even be administered for spinal stenosis or lower back pain.

Whilst the above can be effective with chronic pain management they also bring their own added risks to the table, especially if you take them over the long term. The side effects of some medications can be worse than the actual ailment you're trying to treat. You could even become addicted to these medications. Man-made chemicals are rarely as good as nature's own products.

CBD oil could provide a great natural alternative. In 2008, a study investigated the efficacy of cannabinoids other than THC in pain management. It showed that participants tolerated painkillers containing cannabinoids very well, with minimal side effects and without the issue of long-term toxicity. In addition, when CBD, was combined with opioids, the effect was even more pronounced, and many researchers believe that this is the breakthrough for future in palliative care.

Managing anxiety

Severe anxiety can prove debilitating and drive suffers to extremes as they attempt to avoid any anxiety-producing situation. Unfortunately, most of the current treatment options are less than ideal. These medications are very hard on the body. Some people turn to therapists with varying degrees of success. An improperly trained therapist can make a bad situation worse.

CBD oil has exhibited some success at managing anxiety. The anxiolytic effect of THC is documented in many different studies and when it is combined with other cannabinoids, such as CBD, it can provide relief. The exact way CBD works to treat anxiety has not yet been ascertained. However, a preliminary study published in 2013 in the *International Neuropsychopharmacology Journal* has set the foundation for more research in the future to show that CBD could be a great treatment for anxiety and for depression in many patients.

This is especially true for those who are dealing with situations that have not improved using more traditional methods. CBD oil is very effective in calming the individual down — to decrease excitement and worry. I have experienced reduced anxiety and stress levels through taking CBD oil and taking other measures like watching what I eat and drink along with exercise and being selective about who I spend time with.

Insomnia

One of the most popular uses of CBD is to help with insomnia. Research has shown a significant relationship between CBD, the central nervous system, the endocannabinoid system, and various neurotransmitters in the brain. Even though the CBD part of the plant is not intoxicating, it is able to positively affect your mood. It can also act on the serotonin receptors in the brain, can regulate the GABA regulators that are involved in anxiety, and much more.

There are other products on the market to help with insomnia, but again often these have a lot of bad side effects and require the introduction of unnatural chemicals to your body. With the help of natural CBD, you can deal with insomnia without having to worry about all the usual side effects that often come with other products.

Overall CBD has helped me sleep a bit better although I prefer not to take my oil any time after 8pm. Any later than this and I can sometimes feel a bit foggy for the first half of the following morning. It didn't always happen however taking before 8pm works for me. I believe CBD should be considered as a temporary fix in this regard until your anxiety or stress is reduced to the point that you can sleep soundly.

Various autoimmune disorders

It is also possible to use CBD oil to help manage a variety of autoimmune disorders. This can be ideal for people who are dealing with these disorders and who have not had success with conventional medications. Autoimmune disorders can be dangerous and difficult to deal with. Those with autoimmune disorders may need to change their diets, their lifestyles, and even go on medication that is potentially harmful and doesn't really seem to do much to make them feel better.

CBD oil has a singular mechanism of naturally reducing inflammation in most patients without the usual unwanted effects.
This could change the we deal with autoimmune diseases in the long term. Sufferers can take CBD toil and see a vast, almost immediate, improvement.

Acne

While this one may not seem as important as some of the others on the list, it is still another health benefit to consider. Acne is a common skin problem that touches almost everyone at one point or another. More than nine percent of the population suffer from it on a regular basis and find that other treatments just do not work.

There are a lot of reasons for acne, including genetics, inflammation under the skin, bacteria, and an overproduction of sebum in the body. Based on some recent studies, it is possible that CBD oil could treat acne mostly due to the oil's ability to reduce inflammation. CBD is effective at reducing the amount of sebum production in the body, which can mean less acne as well.

One study found that CBD could prevent the sebaceous gland cells from secreting excessive sebum while also preventing the activation of "pro-acne" agents like inflammation cytokines. Another study had some similar findings and concluded that CBD may be a safe and efficient way to treat acne, especially if you have tried other methods without success. CBD oil could either be consumed orally or even applied locally to treat Acne.

Antibacterial

There have been several studies demonstrating how CBD oil exhibits antibacterial properties. One such study, performed at the Italian Piemonte University and later published in 2008, implied that all types of cannabinoids help the immune system fight bacteria.

Even though all of cannabinoids are effective at helping with this, it seems there are five cannabinoids, including CBD, that the study focused on because of their antibiotic resistant properties. Considering that a lot of people are overusing antibiotics and are now resistant to them, it is nice to think there may be a healthy and effective alternative with so many variations of CBD available then one shouldn't need to worry about building up a tolerance and for CBD to one day become ineffective.

One of the biggest reasons some people choose to go with this treatment is because the chemicals contained in CBD reduce inflammation in the body. CBD enhances bone growth, making them stronger and more resistant to inflammation, osteoporosis and other disorders.

There are even some studies, most notably the ones from the University of Tel Aviv, that discovered rats given CBD supplements recovered from fractures up to 40 percent faster compared to those who did not take the supplement. CBD oil may provide relief for these conditions and accelerate the healing process.

Headaches

Most of those who use CBD oil for headaches have already been dealing with this debilitating pain for a long time. They may have tried a lot of different medications throughout the years and are still not seeing any meaningful benefits. Regular headaches negatively impact quality of life and can limit the activities in which they participate.

CBD oil works with the transmitters in the brain to alleviate pain. CBD can be very effective even if other treatments or medications have not worked in the past. If you are tired of dealing with headaches and nothing else seems to work for you, then it may be time to try some CBD to see if that can give you a little bit of relief. I have had some success with treating tension headaches with CBD.

It's strange though that CBD wasn't as effective at treating a headache and accompanying sore bones which I experienced through suffering a nasty cold. I wound up taking CBD and paracetamol together which worked fine without any adverse effects. On another occasion the same CBD brand lifted my headache albeit I did not have an accompanying cold on that occasion.

Eating disorders

In some cases, cachexia and anorexia patients can use CBD and cannabis as an effective and safe treatment. Cachexia is a severe disorder that involves a dangerous amount of weight loss. This is a bit different than some of the other eating disorders that you may encounter because rather than the patient purposely trying to lose the weight, this dangerous weight loss is brought on by some sort of disease, such as Alzheimer's (where the patient may forget to eat), cancer, or AIDS.

In 2011, a study in Germany involving over 100 people proved that patients who were on a placebo were able to lose about 80 percent more weight each week compared to those who received a cannabinoid cocktail. This shows that the CBD oil may be able to prevent weight loss or help you to keep on or gain weight if needed.

Additionally, CBD oil can be used as a form of treatment for those who are suffering from a variety of eating disorders, including anorexia nervosa. While gaining weight, the CBD user also benefits from the calming and mental-improvement qualities of the oil.

Tourette's Syndrome

Tourette's Syndrome affects about one percent of the population. The cause of this disorder is unknown, but while more and more people are diagnosed with this disorder each year, most treatment options are lacking. According to Kristen R. Muller-Vahl, M.D., current treatments are unsatisfactory, which has led to more interest in using cannabis and other holistic treatments.

Muller-Vahl describes two clinical studies conducted in 2002. One of these studies involved giving 12 patients one dose of THC. Two weeks later, they were given a placebo. Seventy-five percent of the participants reported positive effects from the first round.

The second study had 24 participants, all of whom were affected by tics from TS. With this study it was reported that THC was able to reduce tics in patients. in addition, neither study showed that there were serious adverse effects to taking cannabis for this disorder. Muller-Vahl suggests that when the major Tourette's Syndrome drugs do not work for patients, then using CBD can be an effective treatment. CBD has reduced the number of ticks in my friend's young son.

PTSD

You can also use CBD oil to help deal with symptoms of PTSD. Most sufferers of this use this oil to self-medicate, so studies on it are not as prevalent as for other disorders. Many of those who have PTSD find it difficult to cope with the unpleasant and intense symptoms. Issues like nightmares, anger, hyperarousal, sleep problems, and intrusive memories and thoughts are common and can interfere with the daily functioning of these individuals.

Taking one of the suitable strains of CBD can help provide quick relief from these symptoms. It can get rid of the anxiety and help the sufferer relax. It may not address the root of the problem and those suffering from PTSD will need to take other treatment actions, however CBD can help to relax the patient. Once in this more beneficial relaxed state, patients are in a better position to be treated with other therapies and methods either alongside of or without cannabis.

Period pain

It is believed that CBD can even help with monthly period pain. A 2002 review described tonics (made as early as 2000 BC) that were made from beer, mint, saffron, and hemp seed and then given to women to help ease their pain during difficult childbirth. In 1596, a medical text from China listed that this a good way to ease symptoms that women experienced during menstruation. It is said that Queen Victoria used the herb to receive relief from painful cramping and it was common for Victorian doctors to prescribe this as well.

Today, even with the issues of legality of the herb in most of the world, women are still turning to CBD to self-treat problems they have with the womb. This includes those who use it to help with period cramps, pregnancy complications, bloating, and more. CBD has also been shown to help some women deal with the symptoms of menopause by helping to balance hormones.

Boosting athletic performance

This one really caught my attention. There is evidence that CBD can be used to improve athletic performance. In fact, it can be viewed as a tool for use in sports medicine. There are not many available studies on the subject at this moment however there is a lot of anecdotal evidence stating how CBD increases concentration, confidence, and stamina during athletic activities.

Cannabidiol can be used to boost any kind of athletic performance and long-distance runners are a good example of how this can work. Many long-distance runners have shared how CBD has helped them to have more endurance and positive mental focus while training. Snowboarders and skiers talk about how it can help them to concentrate and lose their fear and anxiety when they are on the slopes.

In addition, heavy weightlifters mention how CBD lessens the amount of stress that they feel when working on a heavy lift. CBD talk has also made it onto the football field. Many believe that it helps players cope with off-field pain better than taking traditional painkillers and that it could help treat traumatic brain injury.

The health benefits were of interest to me. I have found that the general feeling of wellbeing that can be acquired with CBD has a knock-on effect of other areas including fitness. Cycling and weightlifting for me were areas where I noticed an improvement at times while taking the oil as part of a balanced diet and solid lifting routine. When our bodies are in balance, hormone production is improved which can aid us in lots of ways, not just fitness.

Hepatitis C

There is some research suggesting that cannabidiol could offer therapeutic benefits to those who are suffering from HCV and other diseases of the liver. Cannabinoids can bind and influence the CB1 and CB2 receptors in the endocannabinoid system. The CB2 is responsible for reducing inflammation in the body and can be beneficial on alcoholic fatty liver, liver injury, regeneration, fibrosis, and hepatic inflammation.

Patients have found some success with taking cannabis to help treat the symptoms they experience with Hepatitis C and the nausea that can come from some of the treatments of this disease.

Fibromyalgia

Fibromyalgia sufferers may be able to get more relief from medical marijuana than they can from any of the three prescription drugs approved by the FDA. Medical marijuana is as the name suggests. It is marijuana which has been medically prescribed by a doctor to treat an illness. According to the National Institutes of Health, there are roughly five million Americans who suffer from fibromyalgia, a condition that can include symptoms such as lack of sleep, depression, headaches, fatigue, and deep tissue pain. Many respondents to a survey from the National Institutes of Health say that they have tried at least one prescription medication for their symptoms, and quite a few had tried all three.

Sixty to 70 percent of patients agreed that these prescriptions did not work and that the limited relief did not warrant the side effects.

However, 62 percent of those who tried cannabis to treat their symptoms said that it was very effective, and another 33 percent said that it helped a little. Compared to prescription medications where most people saw no relief, only five percent of those who tried cannabis said that it did not work.

Schizophrenia

There is currently an experimental cannabis drug used to treat schizophrenia. This drug was developed by GQ Pharmaceuticals Plc, a UK-based business, and was found to be superior to a placebo in mid-stage trials. The drug, cannabidiol, was tested on 88 patients, all of whom experienced schizophrenia but had not responded to anti-psychotic medication in the past.

During the trial, the patients continued to take their medications while some received a placebo and other received the cannabidiol. This study found that those who took the cannabis experienced fewer episodes of schizophrenia compared to those that took the placebo. GW has plans to test this drug on other health-related issues including pain from cancer and epilepsy.

CBD in mother's breast milk

Emerging research shows that cannabinoids found in the breast milk are important to the development and growth of the human infant. These chemicals can help to jumpstart the appetite of the baby because the mother produces cannabinoids naturally, which ultimately promote the healthy development in the baby.

Studies have shown that two endocannabinoids, anandamide and 2-arachidonyl glycerol, are both found in the human embryo. In the beginning, the anandamide works to help regulate the appetite and one's pleasure and reward systems. It begins in low concentrations in the embryo and then will slowly increases until the baby is mature. The 2-arachidonyl glycerol works the opposite way.

The baby, when born, will not produce CBD on their own. Babies rely on the mother's milk to provide them with this chemical to keep their appetite up and to aid in their development. If the baby has trouble gaining weight and doesn't have much of an appetite, the mother may want to talk to her doctor about including some CBD oil in her diet. This chemical would then be passed on to the baby through the milk and could help the baby to increase appetite and in turn, gain more weight.

CBD for beauty and anti-aging

Many have decided to start using CBD to help fight the effects of aging and to make them look younger and more vibrant. CBD oil is full of great antioxidants and vitamins that can protect your body from the harmful effects of free radicals. It can even protect you from the sun. If your body is exposed to too many of the above, over time your skin will start to show it.

Using a topical form of CBD can help to keep the skin looking good. The high concentration of vitamin A in the oil, which is crucial to the growth and differentiation of skin cells, helps your skin look amazing. In addition, the vitamin D inside the oil combines with vitamin A to prevent the skin from getting flaky and dry. It is an extremely good natural moisturizer.

Other benefits

Because of the rising popularity of CBD, many new studies are being conducted to explore how multi-functional CBD oil can be and how much it can do to keep the human body healthy. While many people may still be worried about trying out this treatment because of its association with cannabis, I suspect it won't be long before it becomes more of a staple in our culture. Some of the other benefits you could receive with the use of this treatment includes:

- Antipsychotic effects: Some studies are suggesting that using CBD could help people who are suffering from schizophrenia and some other mental disorders. It can do this by reducing the psychotic symptoms of the sufferer.

- A treatment for substance abuse: CBD has been shown to modify the circuits in the brain that are closely related to drug addiction. In rats, CBD reduced dependence on morphine while also reducing heroin seeking behavior.

- Anti-tumor effects: In animal and test tube studies, CBD has demonstrated the ability to stop tumors. It can even help to prevent the spread of various cancers like lung, colon, brain, prostate, and breast.

As you can see, for some people there are a ton of potential health benefits with CBD oil. Whether you need help with an autoimmune disorder, want to improve your heart, have issues with headaches, and more, you could find that adding CBD to your lifestyle could make a profound difference in how you think and feel.

Are there any side effects?

Yip there can be as I document further in the chapter 'CBD and me'. Under normal conditions however most people have reported zero side effects although it's important to note that some people may experience some side effects albeit relatively minor in nature. If a person feels any of these side effects, they should consider reducing their dose or perhaps switch CBD brands to see if this makes a difference. Typical side effects include:

- Light headedness due to low blood pressure: Taking too much CBD oil for your condition can result in a lower blood pressure. This will usually happen soon after taking the CBD. This is a temporary side effect, however if you are already taking medication for your blood pressure, you be exercising some caution here and stick to your recommended dose of CBD. Again, always consult with your doctor before you get started using CBD.

- Fatigue: CBD should make you feel awake and full of energy, however a dose which is too high can sometimes cause drowsiness. If you start to feel drowsy when taking your CBD, then obviously you should not drive or operate machinery etc. The drowsiness should pass in a couple of hours. Consider reducing your dose. If it continues then perhaps try another brand.

Remember that these side effects are not going to be the same for everyone. Some people will experience mild cases of these effects, but most people take CBD oil and (as long as they stay within the dosage that is correct for them) will be perfectly fine. As always listen to your body and be careful, albeit this is the same advice you would follow no matter what kind of new supplement you use.

The truth is that CBD will be highly effective at treating some people and not others since everyone is different. Again, just keep in mind that trial and error is expected until a person finds what works for them.

More about THC in CBD

Now earlier on in the book we discussed how THC is the psychoactive compound that gets you high. CDB oil requires to have a THC content of 0.3% or less to remain legal as this is such a small amount of THC that it will go undetected in the body and the person will not feel high from it.

THC in small doses can however have a positive effect alongside CBD in the management of some ailments. Because of this some plants are specifically designed and engineered or cross bred to have the desired qualities to treat specific ailments.

So far these have been very effective and successful however we need to re-emphasize that THC needs to be less than 0.3% in most countries, to remain on the right side of the law. This is one of the current issues with the laws around CBD. We know that a CBD with more than the allowed 0.3% of THC can be very good at treating epilepsy amongst other things. Now you could easily buy such a product with good intentions however if you live in a country where the THC content needs to be legally under 0.3% then you are breaking the law and the penalties could be harsh.

Below are some very general examples of how CBD could be consumed by various methods. Note that some conditions can be treated using CBD with a higher THC content than 0.3%.

Help increase appetite in cancer patients: 2.5 milligrams of THC by mouth with or without 1 mg of CBD for six weeks.

For chronic pain: 2.5-20 mg CBD under your tongue daily for 1 month.

Help manage epilepsy: 200-300 mg of CBD by mouth daily.

Help with movement problems associated with Huntington's disease: 10 mg per kilogram of CBD by mouth daily for six weeks.

Treat sleeping disorders: 40-160 mg CBD by mouth.

Manage multiple sclerosis symptoms: Cannabis plant extracts containing 2.5-120 milligrams of a THC-CBD combination by mouth daily for 2-15 weeks. A mouth spray might contain 2.7 milligrams of THC and 2.5 milligrams of CBD at doses of 2.5-120 milligram for up to eight weeks. Patients typically use eight sprays within any three hours, with a maximum of 48 sprays in any 24-hour period.

Help treat schizophrenia: 40-1,280 mg CBD by mouth daily.

Treat glaucoma: a single CBD dose of 30-40 mg under your tongue. Doses greater than 40 mg may increase eye pressure.

Points to remember:

- CBD can be used to effectively treat a host of ailments and can also be used as a health tonic.
- There are no real short, long term or side effects however be careful if you have low blood pressure. If you do experience side effects, then stop then reduce your dose.
- THC content can be higher than 0.3% to treat some ailments although there is a legal aspect to consider here.
- Other cannabinoids are also beneficial to us.

Chapter 4:

How to take your CBD oil?

Taking CBD for your health is a breeze. There are a few different methods you can use. The method you choose will really be down your personal preferences and how soon you want the CBD to take effect. Try experimenting to see what works best for you. Some of the options you have for ingesting CBD include:

Tinctures

The most common way to use CBD is a tincture. Compared to the other products, tinctures are considered the purest application of CBD because the manufacturers do not do any separate processing of the oil. Some brands add flavoring to the tinctures. This simply makes it more palatable for consumers to take and it doesn't change the purity of the product. CBD oil in its natural form has an earthy nutty taste which I didn't find unpleasant at all.

To take you simply put a few drops either on or under the tongue. The biggest issue with using a tincture is that they get messy if you spill any of the drops. For this reason, some people are not entirely comfortable using tinctures however I use it myself and I have no problems with it. You just need to be careful not to spill any because being an oil it can easily stain furniture or clothes.

A tincture is most effective if you do not swallow all the liquid straight away. It's beneficial to ingest as much of it as you can sub-bilingually. To do this try placing the drops along the cheeks or under the tongue and then leave them there, without swallowing, for as long as you can for the best results. This gives the CBD time to absorb into your bloodstream before the rest goes through your digestive tract. You should start to feel the effects within 10 minutes, and they'll last for 3-4 hours. A 30ml tincture contains around 720 drops of oil.

Concentrates

A CBD concentrate is the strongest dosage of CBD. They could contain up to 10 times the concentration of CBD compared to other similar CBD products. Some people appreciate the convenience that the concentrate offers, particularly those on higher daily doses of CBD.

CBD concentrate typically is not flavored and the natural CBD flavor is slightly intensified making it bit less palatable for some users. Some newcomers to CBD have also reported being a bit turned off by the syringe shape as they find it bit intimidating.

For the most part, the CBD concentrates are popular with customers. Concentrates have a high potency and are easy to take so you can get your dosage quicker. To take a CBD concentrate, simply place it under your tongue and along the cheeks and then let it slowly dissolve. Just like the tincture method you should feel the effects within 10 minutes, and they will last for 3-4 hours. A user should be mindful of the high strength of the concentrate and not take too much.

Capsules

Another option you can choose is a CBD capsule. This one is often considered the easiest method to use because you simply take the CBD as a supplement, just like you would take your daily multivitamin. The capsules are easier to take compared to the other two methods, and if you are already taking other supplements, you can easily add the CBD pills to this daily regimen.

The capsules offer between 10 and 25mg of CBD. Since each capsule already offers a set amount, you will find this is one of the easiest ways to keep track of how much you are taking. The pills can sometimes present issues if you want to change your dosage. Some people get around this by using capsules along with some other types of CBD products, like a tincture, so that they can adjust and control the amount they take.

There's no denying that capsules are convenient. You just take one, or as many as needed, with water each day to get the desired dosage and results. You should feel the effects of capsules anywhere between 30 minutes to 2 hours as they must travel through your digestive tract. Effects will last for 3-4 hours.

Topicals

It is becoming more common to see CBD in topicals, such as lip balms, salve, and lotions. These products deliver great natural anti-aging skin benefits. Topicals help with a whole host of things such as a cancer treatment, anti-wrinkle treatment, psoriasis, acne, inflammation, and chronic pain.

If you decide to use topical products, look out for the keywords on the product label. Look for *micellization, encapsulation*, or *Nanotechnology* of CBD. This shows that the solution can carry the CBD through your dermal layers to provide relief, rather than just keeping it on the skin. Using the CBD infused topical layers are meant to help more with joint or skin-related issues.

To use topicals that are infused with CBD, just follow the same rules as you would with other body care products. Use it as necessary on the area of need. You can apply it generously to any area of the body and effects should start to be felt within around 15 minutes and last 3-4 hours. I tried using topicals to shave with and it was very effective. It left my skin feeling great.

Sprays

Most CBD users stay away from the sprays because they have the weakest concentration compared to the other types of CBD products. Most concentrations found in these sprays will range from 1 to 3mg, which is not very high. And when you compare them to the other oral products, it can be tricky to measure the exact amount that you take each day because the sprays are inconsistent.

Sprays are convenient and easy to carry around – especially on the road. If you are traveling, it is much easier to spray some of the CBD into your mouth compared to fiddling about with a concentrate or a tincture. You may need to spray a few times to get any effects though because the concentration and volume of product per spray is so low in these sprays.

To use, just spray one serving of the bottle straight into your mouth. Each type of spray will be different, so look for the serving size on the label and use this as a rough guide. The serving size will usually be somewhere between two and three sprays. You could use these sprays as needed or to top up your tinctures or concentration method while on the move. The effects should take place within 10 minutes and last for 1-2 hours.

Vapes

Some people choose to ingest their CBD oil through vapes. Based on some reviews from those who have tried it, ingesting the CBD through vape oil seems to have lower effects compared to some of the other methods that we have discussed. However, others say that vaping has fewer drawbacks and is more convenient than compared to taking CBD orally. The effects should take place within 10 minutes and last for 1-2 hours.

Edibles

For some people, going with the options above can prove to be less than ideal. They may need more relief than they can get with a topical solution. Some may not like the taste of the CBD chemical, even if there are added flavors to the product. They may not be interested in trying other methods. Anyway, sometimes you just want to try something a bit different and see how it works. Long term users may just fancy a bit of variety and adding CBD to food and drink can be a worthwhile routine.

For these individuals, edibles may be the best option. Edibles are any type of food or beverage containing the oil. You can technically add the CBD to any meal or snack that you make. This helps to mask the flavor and make consumption a bit more interesting and varied. Many people like to add the oil to a nice dessert, but you can also go with other options, even beer, wine and cocktails.

Later, there are several different recipes to try if you want to consume your CBD as an edible. These include options for pantry goods, breakfasts, main meals, and desserts and snacks. I chose these recipes because they lend themselves well to CBD plus, they're easy to make and they do taste good. You can mix and match the recipes that you want to use to get your daily dosage.

Remember that edibles take a bit longer to get the relief. The oil must go through your digestive tract before it absorbs into your bloodstream. This can take up to two sometimes even three hours so clearly it is not as fast as some of the other options that are absorbed more directly, like tinctures or concentrates. But for some people, this is the best option to get their dosage of CBD and it can be fun trying out the recipes. Remember CBD is nutritious, organic and plant based so it will compliment most eating styles and diets.

Other options

The options above are some of the most popular forms of taking CBD oil and most of them can work well in getting your required daily dose. There are a few other options you can choose from including:

- CBD gums
- CBD patches
- Gel pen
- CBD infused water

The only issue with CBD edibles is that unless you are making your own or you make single servings, it can be difficult to accurately determine consistency and potency of servings.

Points to remember:

- CBD can be added to any hot or cold food or drink although extreme heat can destroy the nutrients
- Tinctures and concentrates offer the most efficient method of consumption
- Dosage can be topped up with other methods
- Sprays and Vapes offer the weakest CBD content

Chapter 5

How much CBD oil should I take?

Hmm this is a bit of a grey area and some experimentation is still usually required since we are all different. The FDA will only allow CBD Hemp oil manufacturers to sell CBD oil as a food supplement and not as a medical product or remedy. As such there is currently a lack of scientific data available on exactly how much CBD a person should take in each situation. CBD is however becoming very popular and mainstream now and soon companies will be very keen to show us scientific evidence to support their CBD products. This is of course a good thing because the sooner people are educated and convinced of the merits of CBD the sooner, they can potentially benefit from these oils themselves or at least make an informed choice on whether try CBD oil.

Because of the current food supplement classification of CBD products manufacturers are required to label their products with some form of nutritional and serving size information, like what you would find on food labels in supermarkets or the grocery store.

This has undoubtably caused CBD manufacturers some concern as they've pretty much taken an educated guess at a typical serving size to put on their labels. As such the suggested serving size as shown on these labels should be taken with a pinch of salt (sorry I couldn't resist that.)

What we do know is that so far no one has reported any real adverse effects from taking too much oil. That's encouraging. I myself can personally vouch for this as I had a go at taking more than the recommended dose just to see what happened. All in the name of research and my own curious nature of course. Read what happened later in the book.

OK so with regards to what dose to take what we do have are some tried and tested guidelines which can be followed based on the severity of the condition you are treating and your bodyweight. Incidentally the same rules apply to treating animals with CBD.

Now I appreciate that this sounds a bit rudimentary and it is however do keep in mind that consuming CBD oil for the first time is just like taking any other supplement. Some trial and error are expected, and it is necessity to start with small doses and gradually increase until you find what works best for you. Start by taking one dose in the morning and one in the evening for the first week.

Once you know that it's working for you and your system is used to the oil then consider taking your daily dose in one go at a time that suits you. From this point you can gauge when and how much CBD to take based on your pain levels at various times of the day or night. Just experiment a little and listen to your body-it's always right. You could also perhaps keep a diary to record and monitor your thoughts as you progress.

Right, now let's look at how to get you started. First you need to know how many milligrams of CBD you are taking. Let's say a bottle indicates that 10 drops are one serving size and that serving is 5mg of CBD. In this scenario you could potentially take 20 drops to get 10mg of CBD or 30 drops to get 15mg of CBD and so on.

Below are some examples which you could use as a rough guide to get you started on your CBD journey. Again, please remember to start small then slowly add, tweak and adjust your dosage until you find your sweet spot.

A person with chronic pain who weighs 160lbs may start with a daily dose of 15mg and increase accordingly. Another person weighing 200lbs and who has cancer and is being treated with chemotherapy might start with a daily dose of 25-30mg per day depending on how they feel from day to day.

- For general health, take 2.5 to 15mg of CBD by mouth each day.
- To treat issues with chronic pain, take 2.5 to 20 mg of CBD by mouth each day.
- To treat sleeping disorders, take 40 to 160 mg of CBD by mouth each day.

Some general guidelines to follow include:

- When you first get started with CBD, regardless of the condition you are trying to heal, it is always best to start with the smallest dose possible. You never know how you are going to react to this chemical and since it is so new, you want to be able to learn how your body responds to the supplement before you increase the dosage. Try it out at that dosage for a few days and if you feel that it is not quite doing the job, then add a little more of the CBD to your
regime. As soon as you feel that the dosage is right and is relieving you of the pain or discomfort, then maintain that dose and monitor the situation.

- Pay attention to size and weight of a user. The right dose is going to vary between someone who is small and someone who is bigger. If you are small, such as short or underweight, start out with a very low dose of CBD. If you are a larger person, then you will want to try out a bit more of the oil to see how it goes. With CBD, it is easy to add just a few milligrams to the dosage.

- Talk to a medical professional: If you are dealing with medical conditions, or you are on any type of medication, it is best to talk with your health care professional before you consume the CBD. There are some medications that do not work well with CBD, or which may become less potent when you take CBD and you want to make sure that this does not affect you in a negative manner. A health care professional will be able to answer your questions about CBD and can tell you which doses are the most beneficial based on your personal medical history.

Chart to show dosage relative severity range and bodyweight

SEVERITY RANGE	WEIGHT OF PERSON 31-60 lbs	WEIGHT OF PERSON 60-100 lbs	WEIGHT OF PERSON 100-175 lbs	WEIGHT OF PERSON 175-250 lbs
MILD 1	2mg-4mg +	4mg-6mg +	6mg-8mg +	8mg-10mg +
2	4mg-8mg +	6mg-12mg +	8mg-18mg +	12mg-20mg +
MEDIUM 3	8mg-12mg +	12mg-18mg +	18mg-24mg +	22mg-30mg +

4	12mg-18mg +	18mg-24mg +	24mg-32mg +	32mg-40mg +
SEVERE 5	18mg-30mg +	24mg-40mg +	32mg-60mg +	42mg-60mg +

Chart to show amounts of CBD relative to bottle size

Product Mg	Bottle Size	Drops per bottle	Mg CBD per drop
100 Mg CBD Oil	15 ml	300	.33 mg
300 Mg CBD Oil	15 ml	300	1 mg
600 Mg CBD Oil	15 ml	300	2 mg
900 Mg CBD Oil	15 ml	300	3 mg
1200 Mg CBD Oil	30 ml	600	2 mg
1800 Mg CBD Oil	30 ml	600	3 mg

Points to remember:

- Always consult your Doctor before taking CBD oil.
- There is no scientific data with exact doses available yet.

- Always start with the smallest dose and gradually increase it if need be.

Chapter 6: How to Purchase CBD Oil

Buying CBD oil wasn't quite as simple as I thought it would be. There seems like a million different types and brands of oil on the market. Having such choice is great but it can also be a bit overwhelming with so much to consider before deciding to buy. Before you dive into shopping mode, ask yourself these questions:

- **Why do I want CBD oil?**
  Is it to treat pain or anxiety? Is it for a general health tonic?

- **What strength do I want and how much am I willing to spend?**
  Do you want to start small and test the brands or will you want to buy a larger amount to start?

- **What dosage should I start with?**
  COR Standard is 25mg CBD twice a day, but this is only a suggested serving size. Have you used cannabinoid products before? Are you caring for someone who might desire larger quantities?

- **Do I need products that are discreet?**
  Do you travel frequently, or do you want to have CBD available at work?

- **How many milligrams do I want?**
  Do I want CBD in its rawest natural form or CBD that's more bioavailable?

- **Is cost an issue?** CBD isn't cheap. Buy wisely.

When buying CBD oil there are many important things to consider including the strength and concentration of the oil and the legitimacy of the supplier.

Any legitimate CBD companies will not make any direct medical claims. It is a violation of the Food and Drug Administration DSHEA guidelines to make medical claims about CBD products in the treatment of any medical condition or symptom.

Other crucial aspects to consider are the purity and the volume of CBD oil within the product itself. Let's look at what you need to know to buy the right product for your needs.

10 Things you need to consider

1. Are you getting a high-quality product?

Obviously, it is important that you order high-quality CBD oil if you want to gain the maximum potential health benefits. This market is booming and there are a lot of people trying to get in on it. Many of these companies will provide excellent quality oil to the consumer, but others will just look to make a quick buck in a booming trade. Luckily, there are a few things you can look for to ensure that you are getting the best CBD oil possible.

Some companies now offer products that have been accredited and certified. From growing to packaging, all individual processes can be ISO 9001-certified. This ISO certification aims produce products of quality and consistency. Additionally, the ISO/IEC 17025:2017 Accredited Laboratories Test should ensure the CBD is free off:

- Heavy metals
- Foreign matter
- Pesticides
- Residual solvents from the extraction process
- Bacteria and fungus

2. Consider the source

Hemp that comes from China is a common choice because it usually costs less, allowing suppliers to offer it for less money and a larger profit. If you want high-quality oil, find a supply from Australia, the United States, or Europe. This sometimes results in a higher price, but it is worth it.

It's worth noting that hemp is a bio-accumulator, meaning it can absorb both the good and the bad from the air, water, and soil in which it's grown. You'll want to know that your CBD oil comes from organically grown hemp that can be tracked to its grown source of origin.

Your CBD oil should be free of toxic substances like heavy metals, herbicides or pesticides. Pesticides and herbicides are often used to protect crops against insects, disease, fungi and to control weeds however these same chemicals can also be very harmful to people too.

You should purchase your new CBD from an organic source that can be traced all the way back to the field where it was grown. This will ensure that it is pure and free of foreign substances that might harm you.

3. Petroleum-free processing

The oil's extraction method is very important. A chemical-free, cold CO2 extraction method gets the most CBD possible out of the cannabis plant. It is sometimes more expensive, so some producers will not use this method, but it is important to go with this option because it uses safer solvents and ensure that you get a pure and potent extract. It is also non-toxic and eco-friendly.

4. Check out independent lab results

If you want to make sure that a product is safe and effective to use, check if there are any independent lab results about the product. Not all companies can provide these lab results, but if you can find these, they will give you some reassurance that the CBD is safe to take and higher in quality.

5. A THC level that is lower than 0.3%

The highest quality of CBD oil contains THC levels lower than 0.3%. This ensures that you get all the good effects from the CBD and none of the unwanted ones. You may find some options that are a bit higher and they are probably still pretty good for you. But, if you want the highest quality, try to go with options that keep the THC low which will also comply with the guidelines set out in the Substance Abuse and Mental Health Services Administration (SAMHSA) If there is the possibility of being drug tested at work, or of you operate heavy machinery, or fall into a number of other categories, you may want to keep the THC level to a minimum. You could seek out CBD oil, which is certified to have low levels of, or no, THC in them. Many reputable sellers do offer products that have absolutely no THC in them.

6. Look for the hemp oil extract using the whole plant

Good quality CBD oils use the whole plant. This means that the oil is taken from all the plant, including the stalks, seeds, and stem. It also includes more than just the CBD inside it such as sugars, secondary cannabinoids, flavonoids, and terpenes. These compounds are believed to work well together to heighten the effect that the CBD has on the body. While some manufacturers only offer CBD from certain parts of the plant, the best quality oil is going to include extracts from the whole plant.

7. The concentration of CBD and the total amount of CBD

It's easy for a company to dilute the CBD content to make more money. You should pay close attention to the *concentration* level of the CBD oil you're buying so that you know you're getting what you're paying for. Concentrations of CBD can vary however, a good quality product will have around 250mg to 1,000mg per fluid ounce. As an example, if you were to consider buying a 4-ounce bottle that contained 250mg of CBD, your concentration would be a rather pitiful 62.5 mg of CBD per ounce which would not make it a worthwhile purchase. The concentration of CBD should always be listed on the product. Be wary if it isn't and use this simple formula to quickly work it out for yourself

- Total amount of CBD (in mg)/volume of container (in ounces) = concentration level
- Example: 1,500mg CBD/4-ounce bottle = 375mg/oz. This a bit more like it.

8. How much total CBD is in the product?

This just means how much you're getting in total. Most bottles are labeled with something like, "1,000mg CBD Oil" or "1,000mg Hemp Extract" which means that the container has a total of 1,000mg of CBD in it.

9. Where to find a good supplier

There is a vast number of different products and brands on the market. You could choose to buy from your local dispensary if you have one. Alternatively finding a good online supplier isn't difficult. There are a few things to consider. Are their CBD products being sold legally, with full transparency and accountability? Finding a transparent CBD company is a good first step towards finding an ethical CBD company.

First impressions count so perhaps try contacting them first before ordering. How is there customer service? Do they get back to you when they said they would? Do they sound polite, helpful and knowledgeable? You're looking for a company /supplier that takes accountability seriously, and who very much cares about their customers and the quality of their products.

Also consider the method you want to use when taking the CBD oil. Look at some of the methods we talked about above to help you decide. Some suppliers will offer more than one type of CBD. Knowing the method, you want to use can help to trim the number of suppliers you consider.

Always look at the reviews of a company. CBD oil is becoming increasingly popular and while there are many legitimate companies to purchase from, there are also many people jumping into this market just to make money. They do not necessarily provide a good quality product. If you read through the reviews of any company you are considering, it should not take long to figure out which companies are legitimate and which ones are not.

10. Product cost

Clearly you also want to look at the price of the products. Be careful about the lower priced options. These have usually added things in their mixtures, or they may dilute the oil, so it is barely useful. Compare supplier prices and product quality and shop wisely. No need to rush in. It's best to spend time going over the many various options and prices. As always, you get what you pay for and spending a bit more is justifiable provided you're buying a quality product. Higher quality CBD will be slightly more expensive when it's:

- Organically grown in USA or Europe by a company which is following all rules and laws
- Higher concentrations of CBD which has been extracted using CO_2 method
- Made from premium quality, full spectrum extract, so other that beneficial compounds are also present
- Tested in third-party labs

Something that you should consider is the bioavailability of the product to help you get the best deal. To keep it simple, bioavailability is the strength of the compound when it reaches the site of physiological activity. This is a major factor of how beneficial the CBD product is overall. There are a lot of forms that CBD can be produced in, from ointments, pastes, and suppositories, all with different ways of being administered.

How much does the pure CBD oil cost? Let's say you are thinking about purchasing a bottle of hemp oil that is 10ml but contains

300mg of CBD. If this bottle costs $32, divide this by the 300 to determine the price you are paying per milligram of CBD. This result is $0.11 per milligram for a 3 percent CBD product.

A $194, 10 ml bottle of hemp oil contains 1500 mg of CBD. The price is $0.13 per milligram of CBD.

While the second product contains more CBD, the cost per milligram is higher, so it is not the best deal for you. You can use these calculations to determine if you are getting a good deal. A bigger bottle is not necessarily a better bottle.

Points to remember:

- Always check the product for actual CBD content.
- Compare brands, prices, review, descriptions and the legitimacy of the company and beware of scammers.
- A THC content of 0.3% or less when buying.
- Seek Organic oils with a CO_2 extraction method.
- Check lab results.

Chapter 7: How to Make CBD Oil

The three methods of making CBD oil

Making CBD oil may not suit some people however it's good to know how to make it in case the opportunity presents itself.

There are a few different methods of making CBD oil. The method you choose is going to vary based on the type of CBD oil you want to make and the method that seems the best for you. The three different methods to extract CBD oil from the cannabis plant include:

> The CO2 method. By pushing CO2 through the plant, using low temperatures and high pressures, you will get the CBD in its purest form. Because of the way this method works, it is often seen as the best, as well as the safest, if you want to extract CBD cleanly. This method will help you to remove harmful substances, such as chlorophyll and it doesn't leave a residue.

> Any oil made by extracting CBD in this manner has a cleaner taste compared to the other two methods. It is a lot more expensive compared to the other two methods, which is why some people do not choose to go with the CO2 method.

> The Ethanol method. CBD is sometimes extracted with the help of high-grain alcohol. The biggest issue with this one is that while it proves a bit more cost effective than the other options, if made incorrectly then this method could potentially harm some of the beneficial natural oils that come with CBD, which may make it a bit less effective for treatment in some of the illnesses and diseases. If made with care however then this method will work well.

> The Oil method. This one is growing in popularity, so it is likely that when you purchase CBD, it will have been produced this way. This method involves extraction using a type of carrier oil. There are a few options you can choose from, but olive oil is the most commonly used. The reason this method is so popular is because you get some of the

nutritional value from the carrier oil and it is also safe and free of those unwanted residues that can ruin the oil.

Let's look at an easy and cost-effective method in more detail.

The Ethanol Method.

Ingredients:

- 30g of ground buds (the dried flower heads or buds of the cannabis plant after they have been ground in a grinder or mortar and pestle)
- Grain alcohol or other food-safe, high % alcohol

You will need:

- Medium size glass, ceramic or metal mixing bowl
- Sieve,
- Medium size catchment container
- Double boiler (a set of two pots that are stacked together with space between them)
- Wooden or metal spoon, silicon spatula, funnel, plastic syringe

Time: Around 45 mins

How to make your oil:

Put the ground buds into the mixing bowl and slowly add the alcohol until it covers the buds. Gently stir for 5 minutes. Filter the solution through the sieve and into the catchment container.

Place the remaining residue in the sieve back into the mixing bowl and again add alcohol and stir as before. Then once again, sieve the mixture into the catchment bowl along with your first batch.

Pour the contents of the catchment bowl into the double boiler and gently bring to the boil. Reduce the heat and let it slowly simmer away the alcohol and stir gently for around 15 minutes. to prevent it sticking to the pan. Once all the alcohol has evaporated scrape the pan with the spatula.

Now place some of the concentrated oil into small dark airtight bottles or dosage containers before it cools and becomes thicker. You can use the plastic syringe to do this or use the opposite end of a metal spoon or fork. Olive, coconut or vegetable oil can then be added to the bottle to dilute the mixture.

This last part can be tricky as you want to do this while the concentrated oil is still warm. The quality and strength of your oil will largely depend on the plant used and how well the oil has been produced. This oil can then be consumed or stored.

Chapter 8: Is CBD Oil Legal?

CBD Oil Is Legal in the UK

There's a lot of confusion around CBD law in general. Many people in the UK assume that CBD is illegal. This isn't true. CBD is currently not a controlled substance and there are no restrictions over its use. If the CBD product was produced from one of the 63 industrial hemp strains that have been approved by the EU, it is 100% legal and can be easily bought on the High Street. It's important to observe however, that not all cannabis oil can be used.

"Cannabis oil" in general is still illegal to possess, buy and sell in the UK. Despite this, the law has recently changed to recognize CBD as a form of medicine. So, regarding medicine, CBD is legal provided that the THC content is 0.2% or less. So, while you're not permitted to buy and sell all cannabis oil freely, many people are still able to legally use CBD oil with a maximum THC content of 0.2%, in the UK for medicinal purposes. CBD Hemp oil with less than 0.2% THC can be sold as a food supplement.

Is CBD Oil legal in the USA?

OK now it gets a bit tricky to explain so we'll try to keep it as simple as possible. While it's true that CBD is legal in all 50 states, there are some situations when it isn't legal. The differences between legal and illegal will depend on several key factors determined by the state in question. The common theme across all states is that to be legal the CBD must come from hemp with a low THC content and not from marijuana which clearly has a much higher THC content.

Is Marijuana-Derived CBD legal?

In some states, marijuana CBD with a high THC content is completely legal, while in others, it is illegal, but in most states, it's a mixed bag with each state having its own CBD laws, which it seems, is in a constant state of change. Canada has completely legalized marijuana in all forms.

On top of this there are some states where hemp-derived and marijuana-derived CBD are legal, which may mean that in time other states may follow suit.

Marijuana and hemp are currently legal for recreational and medicinal use in Alaska, California, Colorado, Maine, Massachusetts, Nevada, Oregon, and Washington. You can legally use CBD in any form without a prescription in these states.

At the time of writing there are 46 states (including the 8 states mentioned above) where CBD is legal with a prescription for medicinal usage. Although CBD usage is legal in these states, the law varies from state to state, with 17 states having specific legislation for the THC-levels in CBD and the conditions being treated with CBD.

The 17 states are Alabama, Florida, Georgia, Indiana, Iowa, Kentucky, Mississippi, Missouri, North Carolina, Oklahoma, South Carolina, Tennessee, Texas, Utah, Virginia, Wisconsin, and Wyoming.

There are 29 states fully legalize the Medical use of all CBD products derived from either hemp or Marijuana are: Alaska, Arizona, Arkansas, California, Colorado, Connecticut, Delaware, Florida, Hawaii, Illinois, Maine, Maryland, Massachusetts,

Michigan, Minnesota, Montana, Nevada, New Hampshire, New Jersey, New Mexico, New York, North Dakota, Ohio, Oregon, Pennsylvania, Rhode Island, Vermont, Washington and West Virginia. Additionally, the territories of Guam and Puerto Rico also allow the use of CBD products on medical grounds.

Prior to buying any CBD product in these states (aside from the 8 mentioned above) you need to have a medical prescription issued by a certified medical doctor. Each state has a concentration of THC it allows to be present in a CBD product, with the percentage ranging from 0.3% – 8%. If you are in any of these states, it is vital to be aware of the state's current laws towards CBD.

Is CBD illegal in any states?

We have discussed 46 states where Marijuana-derived CBD is legal at various levels, however there are also 4 states where Marijuana-derived CBD is completely illegal.

These states are Idaho, Kansas, Nebraska and South Dakota. Although marijuana-derived CBD is legal in these states, the laws are still a bit foggy, so there are businesses selling CBD, and patients considering using CBD in these states should be cautious and careful when considering using CBD products. Always check on the status of the stated laws as they will likely change over time.

As CBD becomes mainstream, there is every chance that both hemp-derived and marijuana-derived CBD could be completely legal in all 50 states, and possibly in many countries around the world within the next 5 years.

CBD Hemp oil currently legal in these countries.

- Argentina
- Austria
- Belgium
- Belize
- Brazil
- Bulgaria
- Canada
- Chile
- China
- Colombia
- Costa Rica
- Croatia
- Cyprus
- Czech Republic
- Denmark
- Estonia
- Finland
- France
- Georgia
- Germany
- Greece
- Guam
- Guatemala
- Hong Kong
- Hungary
- Iceland
- India
- Ireland
- Italy

- Latvia
- Lithuania
- Luxembourg
- Malta
- Netherlands
- Netherlands Antilles
- Northern Ireland
- Norway
- Paraguay
- Peru
- Poland
- Portugal
- Puerto Rico
- Romania
- Russia
- Slovak Republic
- Slovenia
- South Africa
- Sweden
- Switzerland
- U.S. Virgin Islands
- Uruguay

Points to remember:

- CBD with a THC content of 0.2% is allowed in the UK.
- CBD with a THC content of 0.3% is allowed in most States.
- The laws are being revised and need to be checked regularly for updates.

Chapter 9: CBD and me

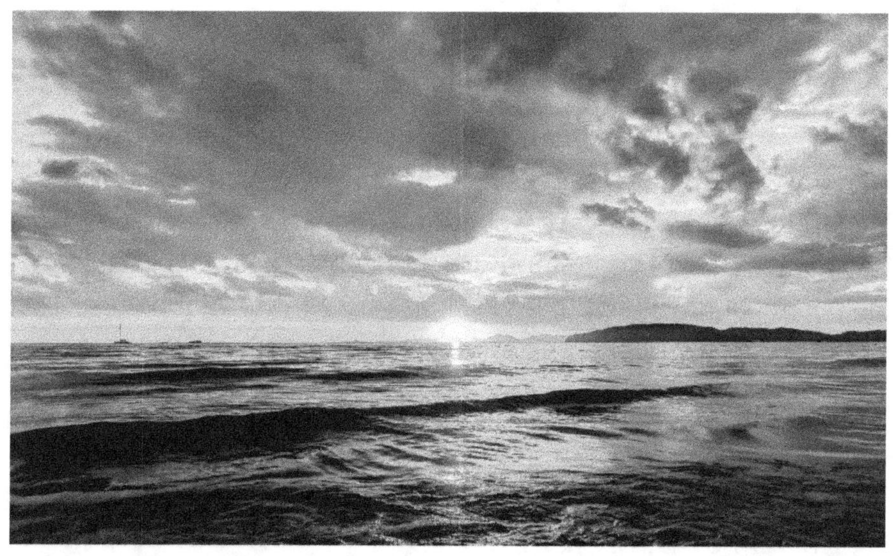

In this chapter I would like to share more of my own personal CBD journey with you so that you can benefit further from my experience, gain some more insight and hopefully save some time and money as well.

I would also like to share some other small health tips that are perhaps a little unconventional but that I've found to be very effective for me. I have successfully managed to naturally bust stress, depression and insomnia and trimmed body fat and gained lean muscle at the same time by consistently practicing some little habits and rituals. These little habits are easy to follow and have served me very well in reaching my health and fitness goals.

Truth be told my decision to experiment with CBD oil suited me perfectly. I have always had an interest in health and fitness and my curious and questioning nature has often been opening to experimenting and trying out alternative therapies and methods to get results. If they're legal of course.

I personally don't see the point in going without the things that give you pleasure. Life's too short for that. To me it's all about balance and moderation. In my experience you can eat and drink whatever you want if you control your portion sizes.

In my workplace they'll say, "What's he doing now?" as I mix various weird and wonderful healthy concoctions. These have generally worked out very well for me over the years. Below are some examples of some methods and habits that have certainly helped me in my quest to be as fit as possible without being obsessed with strict dieting etc.

I've observed that the main reason most people fail to lose bodyfat and get fit is because they don't stick to a routine that works for them long term. After around 2 months of 'healthy eating' they get bored and go back to their old habits. They also are not 100% honest with themselves about what they eat and drink.

Yoyo diets rarely work. Fad diets and strict health regimes are often hard to stick to long term and I personally still want to enjoy wine, beer, curries and crisps and chocolate or whatever else I fancy, whenever I chose and yet still have a decent physique with low bodyfat and some muscle definition. You'll see in the photo of me below that I am no model! I'm not particularly muscle bound, and I perhaps don't have a perfect looking torso but that's the point really. I don't try to be perfect. I'm just an average guy in his mi- forties who wants to enjoy being quite fit while enjoying eating and drinking whatever I please and without ever dieting.

With some little healthy habits here and there, I'm living proof that this can be achievable. CBD has aided me in my efforts to feel better however the main ingredient has been a strong will power and determination. If you truly want something. And I mean REALLY want something you will move mountains to get it. You'll be like a kind of super determined Terminator who will not stop until you get what you want.

It's that sort of mindset that you should adopt to laser focus your mind into making massive changes be it for your health or career or whatever else. I'll add that it gets easier to find that focus once you start to make small changes to feel more positive and healthier in yourself. Feeling positive has several knock-on effects. Once you start to sleep better and deal with nagging pain or anxiety, your positivity will return with a vengeance.

Now I'm not suggesting to you that you do what I do but have a look anyway. This is my usual eating routine. It's not a diet and I never count calories or calculate macronutrients.

- Drink approximately 1 pint of water in the morning before eating or drinking anything. Drink water throughout the day, even if it makes you urinate more frequently.

- Always eat breakfast. My favorite is porridge oats, whole milk, peanut butter, honey, chia seeds, desiccated coconut, flaxseed, blueberries/raspberries and cinnamon. This lot takes less than 4 minutes to make. It's a powerhouse of nutrients and the cinnamon aide's fat loss and lowers blood pressure. You could even add a little chili pepper! Yes, chili pepper! It will ramp up your metabolism and is a great anti-inflammatory. It tastes good too.

- Snack throughout the day with half an avocado, a banana or a handful of unsalted unroasted nuts or full fat natural yogurt which you can add fruit to. I like to add macca powder to mine to help maintain healthy testosterone levels.

- Limit your coffee to 1-2 cups per day.

- Drink green tea. Take omega 3, 6 fish oils during the day. Take ZMA vitamins before bed (Magnesium, Zinc and B6)

- I take 6 drops of 5% CBD oil by tincture orally, placed under my tongue.

- Mix a small amount of apple cider vinegar with coconut oil and the juice of a lemon. Add hot water and a dash of cayenne pepper. This little concoction really helps burn bodyfat and balances your hormones. Seriously.

- Only eat crisps/cakes or biscuits very occasionally as a treat. Same with chocolate. I eat plain chocolate in moderation. The less you eat of these types of foods the less you crave them. The more you eat them the more you want them.

- Try to eat at least some veggies and protein every single day. Cut back a little bit on fast carbs like white bread and pasta. Try having brown bread and whole wheat pasta instead. Eat as much oily fish as you can. I eat tuna and salmon a lot. I also eat well over the recommended amount of eggs. In fact, I drink raw eggs every other day! You should certainly not try this. This goes against every health article or guidance I've ever read however I have been doing this for over 20 years without issue. I only drink free range eggs. Why do I do this? Because for me it's the ultimate convenient protein shake and while it's not particularly easy to drink I do get real benefits from it. I know it sounds a bit disgusting and I guess maybe it is. I blame it on the Rocky films I watched as a kid. Again, I do not advise you to do this. I am simply telling you what honestly works for me. It might not work for you and you could end up ill if you try it. You are much safer eating more cooked eggs perhaps in an omelet or hard boiled.

- This sounds obvious but don't eat unless you are hungry. There's nothing wrong with going without food until you are feeling hungry. Likewise, you don't need to eat everything and leave the plate squeaky clean if you don't want to. Eat until your satisfied and leave the rest if you don't need it. If you know you ate too much over a weekend or a holiday or whatever then reign it back in a little over the next few days. Some people don't seem to know when they've had enough, and they seem to almost 'inhale' large amounts of food each day.

- Walk each day. Or at least move around quite a bit. Don't sit still at a desk all day. Try to exercise in some form or other around 2-3 times a week and integrate it into your lifestyle. Find an activity you really enjoy like cycling, running, swimming, dancing, weights training etc. and make it your habit to do it throughout your life. Do it because you enjoy doing it not because you're 'exercising'. No matter what age you are you should consider doing resistance training i.e. weights training. There are huge benefits to be had here including better sleep, which improves mood, which lessens anxiety, which promotes positivity...you see where I'm going here? Add CBD oil to this little mix and I promise you'll experience big positive changes over time.

- Drink wine or whatever you fancy in moderation. If you do have a heavy drinking session, then drink water throughout the night and drink 2 pints of water before bed and you'll have less of a hangover the next day since a hangover is basically caused by dehydration. I'll admit I love red wine. Perhaps a little too much. I'm very rarely drunk as such, but I do drink a little wine every weekend because I enjoy it. I told you that I was a Scotsman, didn't

I? I do occasionally stop drinking for weeks and months at a time and when I do this, I often see improvements on how I look and feel. Again, moderation is key. Do what you enjoy but do it sensibly and don't do anything too much. Be honest with yourself about exactly what you eat and drink.

A bit more on exercise.

I would like to say to anyone who is suffering from mild to medium stress/anxiety/depression/insomnia that simple exercise can work wonders for you. Cycling, walking or jogging, playing football or gardening are all great examples.

Fresh air and an elevated heart rate are powerful natural anti-depressants. Exercise will produce endorphins and can make you feel on top of the world. High intensity exercise can make you feel like a bit of a superhero. A perfect combination would be outdoor exercise at the weekends and weights training during the week. All subject to your goals and what you wish to achieve of course, be it fat loss or muscle gain or both.

Even simple little changes will all add up over time. Walking to the shops or strolling around the block at lunch time can really make a difference. It doesn't necessarily need to be high intensity, especially not at the start. Often making the initial decision to make a major change can seem like the daunting bit to some people. Be bold and be brave. Tell yourself that you're gonna do this. If you work in an office block like I do, then try taking the stairs rather than the lift. Even start by taking the stairs down at first then attempt to climb up them in the morning. Again, it all adds up.

If you work on the 3rd floor and each floor has two flights of 9 steps, you will burn around 4200 calories per year by just taking the stairs. Or around 6300 calories if you're on the 4th floor. 8300 on the 5th floor and 10400 on the 6th! That's quite a lot don't you think. You will lose fat doing this. My favorite exercise of all time however is cycling.

I just love how off-road cycling makes me feel. It's perfect interval training and zooming down hills is exciting. It's a bit like being a kid again. When you are cycling in the countryside either by yourself or with friends you can experience a physical and spiritual uplift that is very powerful on your mind and body. It can destroy stress or at least make it much more manageable. It will help you sleep better and vastly improve your mood. You might consider giving cycling a try for yourself.

Remember that fitness and wellbeing is 80% nutrition. Notice I never said diet. Get your own nutrition and exercise sorted out and I promise you that you will sleep better and naturally reduce anxiety and depression and you will feel mentality and physically supercharged.

The benefits of exercise cannot be overemphasized. CBD has helped me here because it has made me feel calm and helped me sleep which has aided my recovery after exercise. Faster recovery means getting fitter quicker. You could say that the benefits I've experienced from CBD have had a knock-on effect on other areas.

Years of training in Bruce Lees brutal martial art Jeet Kune Do while exhilarating at the time, left me with a couple of injuries which occasionally surface as a pain in my right wrist.

We had been training hard as always when I fractured my wrist on the hard floor of the large basement where we trained. It was a very painful experience and I almost let out a Bruce Lee like whoooaaaa! when it happened. CBD oil has helped me deal with this pain when it appears. Just taking my drops in my tincture has helped neutralize the pain along with performing its other little tasks like reducing my anxiety and helping me sleep etc. That's the cool thing about CBD oil. When you find the right brand and take the right dose it helps a few different things at once and it helps your body and mind to help naturally treat these ailments. CBD seems to just help it along which makes sense when you consider how our ECS works.

When these other areas or systems start to help themselves then the need to take CBD in my case lessens because my body is now programmed to be less likely to revert to feeling depressed or anxious. I can now use CBD as a 'top up' every now and then if I feel the need to unless I'm dealing with pain of some sort or if a very stressful situation appears in which case, I'd take CBD to help me deal with it.

We are all only human and stress present itself at any time which is quite normal. It's learning to recognize the signs and dealing with it before it gets out of hand which is very important. The right type of CBD along with a good diet and exercise will help with this.

Oh, one more thing. If you have arthritis or joint inflammation another effective treatment which can be used out-with or alongside CBD oil and cream is something called Golden Paste. It contains Turmeric and Turmeric can work wonders on all sorts of ailments for you and your pets and I suggest you give it a try.

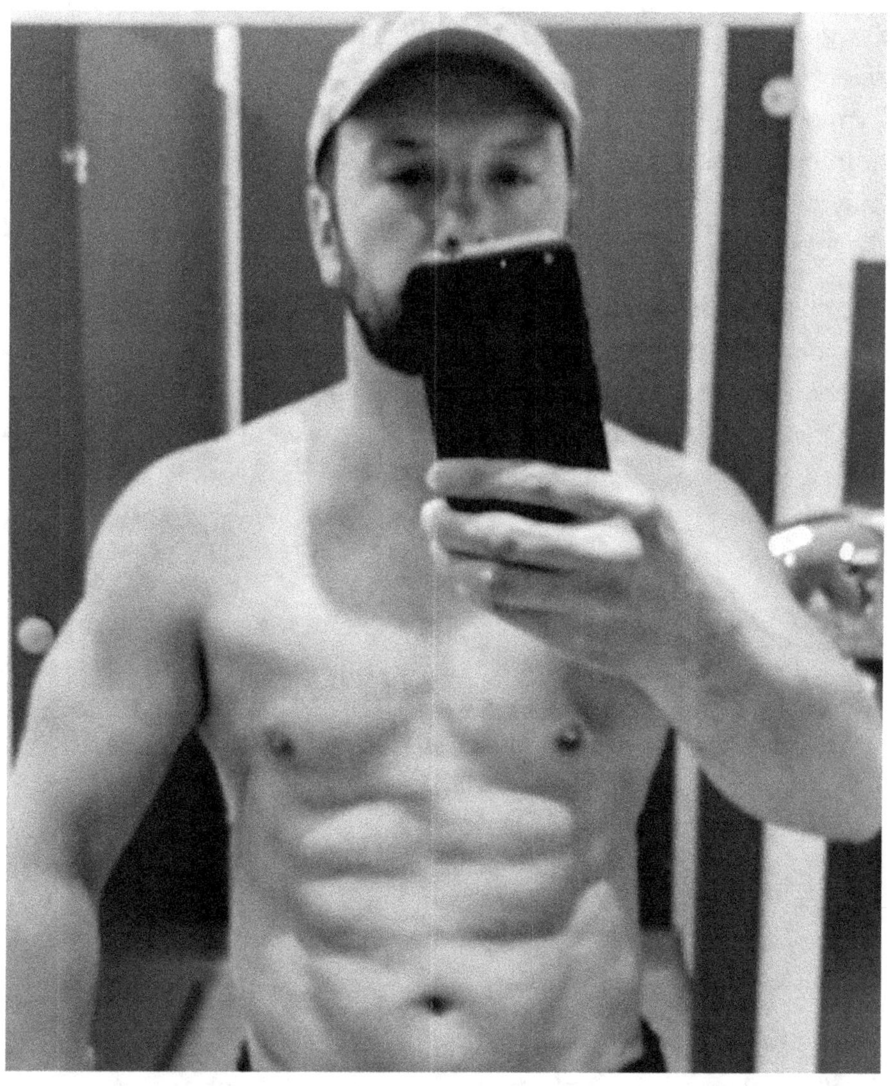

Here's me tensing up my abs in a rather flattering overhead light.
(I never, ever do sit ups or crunches.)

Now let's go back in time a little.

As I've said stress can potentially become serious. It can become a
killer if left unchecked and It can strike anyone at any time. Now

I'm generally quite a relaxed guy who takes things in his stride and deals with life's inevitable ups and downs by working out at the gym or going for long cycles with my friends at the weekends then coming home and eating a curry and having some wine and playing my guitar. This usually does the trick and leaves me feeling up for whatever life will through next at me.

We all have stress from time to time however I can remember two distinct episodes of severe stress in my which were overwhelming and very difficult to deal with. The first was 20 ago years while I was studying for my Degree. My studies coupled with a toxic relationship had left me feeling frazzled and I went to my doctor who prescribed me amitriptyline (an anti-depressant) to help me sleep better.

These small yellow pills did take the edge of my anxiety at times, but they also brought their own little issues too. They made me feel a bit dopey and uninterested and they made me look like I hadn't slept for a week which is odd because they had in fact helped me fall asleep quite quickly.

Strange though that the next day after a full 8 hours shut eye my eyes were quite bloodshot and red. I had a fuzzy chemical hangover feeling. My friend told me that I looked like I'd stuck my face into a jar of pickles!

These pills made me feel a bit weird and I didn't like them. The final straw was when I had a glass of wine with dinner and immediately felt terrible, like I might pass out. This was my own fault as I'd been warned about drinking too much alcohol while taking medications. I didn't think that one small glass was too much though.

I binned these pills and focused hard on meditation and mind training which, coupled with splitting up with Medusa, cycling with my friends, eating curries and drinking the occasional glass of wine, worked out well for me and my stress was reduced enough to complete my studies and get on with my life.

Fast forward to many years later and my second visit to stressed out central materialized through an unexpected mix of cutbacks at work, resulting in daily tensions building up over a period of many months, and a death in my family. This resulted in me taking unpaid leave and travelling around SE Asia with my partner for 6 months which was a truly amazing experience and a great stress buster. But when I returned home and started back at work the stress started to creep back too and I knew I had to do something before it got out of control again. The cycling and the wine weren't quite enough in this instance.

I'd heard about CBD and it immediately appealed to me. My enthusiasm for the subject was a distraction from my stress and I was amazed at the apparent health benefits. It is natural. It has no side effects. It's a bit mysterious and leftfield. It fitted well with my curious nature.

I had bought lots of CBD books and read them one by one however as I said at the start of this book, I was made aware that none of the authors had ever actually taken the oil themselves. I also realized that many of the authors of books and articles on CBD either owned a CBD related company or were affiliated in some way. This gave them a vested interest in shouting CBD's praises.

I wanted the truth, warts and all. I connected to everyone I could through forums and groups all over the World. I wanted to be as educated as possible before diving in myself.

I thought if CBD could help me to relax, take away my wrist pain, concentrate on writing books, help me cope better with work related stress, help me sleep better and help me lose fat and build muscle then I am most certainly keen on giving it a go myself.

My initial CBD intrigue turned into fascination and even an obsession at times. I'd heard stories from a colleague who has been using CBD to treat his healthy 12-year-old pet Labrador for years after the Vet told him that the dog would never walk properly due to a bone problem at birth. The same person has calmed the temper of his angry adolescent son by also giving him a daily CBD capsule.

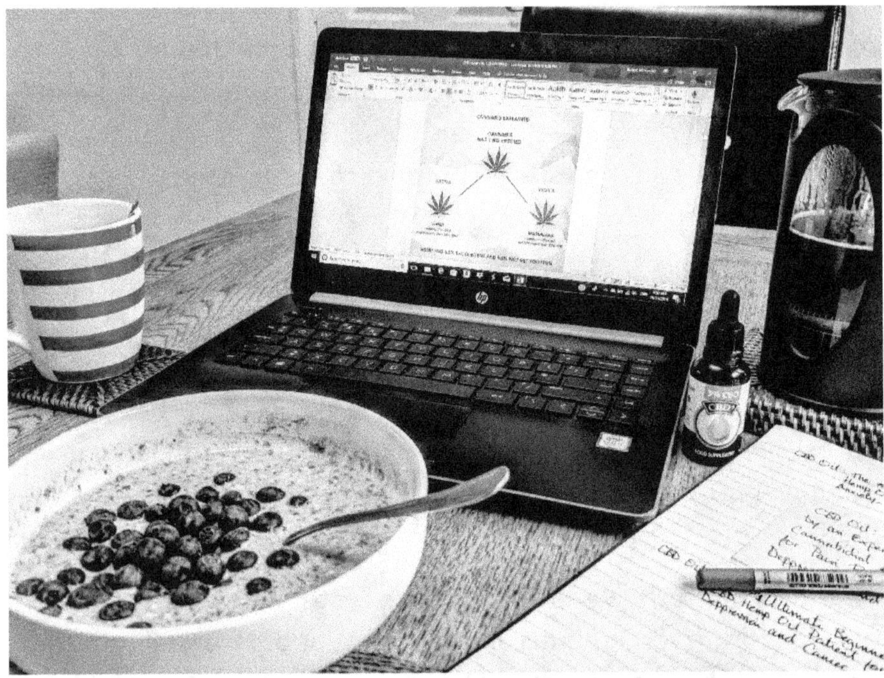

This is what my desk typically looked like while writing this book. Note the super porridge, coffee and CBD tincture all within range.

Around the same time my next-door neighbor who has a been living with a brain tumor started using CBD to manage the symptoms and improve his quality of life. His tumor has shrunk thanks to CBD oil with a <u>higher</u> than the legal 0.3% THC.

It has saved the lives of children with severe epilepsy. It helps animals. It helps stroke victims and people with arthritis.

It could also potentially help my parents. Years of working on roofs has left my Dad with arthritis all over his body. My Mum suffers from insomnia which impact upon her life more than it should. CBD was certainly intriguing to me. It was being hailed as a miracle across the globe and yet some said it was illegal. Or is it? Does it get you high? Does it have side effects? Is it addictive? Is it expensive? What's the best type?

I needed to find out everything I could about CBD oil and then to apply that knowledge and get started with my own CBD journey. Once I decided to try CBD for myself, I just couldn't wait to get started. It was exciting.

I began my research with my usual gusto. I had read everything that I could find, and I had spoken to many people who kindly shared their CBD experience with me. CBD seemed to really change the lives of some people and their pets.

I was excited about the possible health benefits for me and my friends and family. Most people I spoke to have a preferred brand and method of taking the oil. I wanted to try out all the different methods that were available.

I also wanted to know the answers to several key questions that so far no one had been able to answer.

Questions such as, what would happen if I took much more than the recommended dose? Can you mix CBD with other CBD brands, medications or alcohol? Does CBD increase brain capacity and help with concentration and memory? Would it make me fitter and more creative? Would it help me in my work or with learning my guitar?

Without further ado, I dove straight in and decided to get my hands on some CBD as soon as possible.

And then came a big problem. I'm based in Glasgow, Scotland and finding a UK or worldwide supplier was super easy. A quick google search and voila! Lots to choose from. However, finding the **correct** product was proving to be extremely difficult and confusing. Not the straightforward experience that I had read about in various books on the subject.

I knew what I wanted but I still had to spend days just going through details and ingredients of lots of different CBD brands and products.

A lot of suppliers were less than transparent with regards to exactly what they were selling. Some were even misleading in their product descriptions and selling 'hemp oil products' with zero CBD content in them.

These products were stating things like 5% hemp oil but when you studied the contents again there was no CBD to be found. Kind of begs the question, 5% what exactly? Bananas?

The other strange thing was that this product had loads of good reviews and was selling very well indeed. Why? Because it claimed to be a hemp product, it was very cheap compared to the others and packaged well with the little cannabis leaf on the front of a wholesome looking container.

Customers were remarking on how the product was full of omega 3 and 6 essential fatty acids which helped them think clearer and made their hair and nails look shiny. Sure, fatty acids will do this but if that's what you're after then you'd be much cheaper just buying EPA fish oils or by eating more oily fish like salmon or sardines or eat more avocado in your diet.

Lesson one is make sure you're buying CBD oil with CBD in it. If a description is ambiguous then move on. After all there's plenty to choose from.

It's true that the effects of CBD can vary from person hence why experimenting is recommended however I suspect that some suppliers are taking advantage of the current market conditions and selling snake oil rather than CBD oil. Just be very cautious when buying.

Here is an example of the type of product description that you can expect to see online if you're looking for tinctures. When you see a product that you might like you need to delve deeper to make sure it's got what you need.

Below is a completely factitious example of a more honest product and description that you might see. Let's call it Browns Hemp Oil. Again, this is made up. Any similarity to currently available products is completely coincidental. This is just to give you an idea of what to expect and what to look for.

Browns Hemp Oil 1000mg-Organic CBD Hemp Oil for Pain and Stress Relief, Improved Mood, Better sleep, Skin Care (1000mg, 33.3mg per Serving x 30 Servings) $29.99

Product description

Browns CBD Hemp Oil Extract Supports:

- Omega 3 and Omega 6 Supplementation
- Rest and Relaxation*
- Anxiety Relief*
- Cortisol Manager*
- Quality Sleep Patterns*
- Inflammation and Joint Pain Relief*
- Nourishes Hair and Skin*
- Immune, Limbic, Neurogenic System Support*

* These statements have not been evaluated by the Food and Drug Administration. This product is not intended to diagnose, treat, cure, or prevent any disease.

Directions: Shake and squeeze 1-2 servings (1ml or 30 drops per 33.3mg serving) under tongue. Hold for 60 sec before swallowing. Use 1-3 times daily and consistently. Store cool.

Browns Blend:

Here at Browns Hemp Oil we are proud to use a full spectrum oil that includes the natural terpenes and antioxidants present in the hemp plant. Our products include all the phytonutrients present in the industrial hemp plant to give you the full effect of hemp oil. No artificial sweeteners, preservatives or pesticides.

Why buy Browns?

We're Scotland based and use only organically grown hemp from certified Scottish hemp farms. Our hemp is extracted through a state-of-the-art clean CO2 process that leaves nutrients intact without using harmful solvents, and everything is tested for potency and safety.

Purchase with Confidence:

Our product is non-psychoactive with a THC content of 0.2%, and federally legal in all 50 states as it is derived from industrial hemp. We offer a full guarantee - if you are unhappy with any of our products, simply send it back within 30-days and we'll refund your order. Your statutory rights are unaffected.

Important information
Safety Information

Check with your doctor before ingesting any herbal supplements, consumption of herbal ingredients may cause allergies in certain individuals. If you have a known medical condition, you should consult with a healthcare professional before using this or any dietary supplement. If you have a history of allergies to herbal ingredients, do not consume this product. If pregnant, breastfeeding, or on a prescribed medication, consult your physician before use.

Legal Disclaimer

Browns Hemp Oil and these statements have not been evaluated by the Food and Drug Administration. This product is not intended to diagnose, treat, cure, or prevent any disease.

Statements regarding dietary supplements have not been evaluated by the FDA and are not intended to diagnose, treat, cure, or prevent any disease or health condition.

Ingredients

CBD 5% Hemp Seed Oil, Fractionated Coconut Oil, Peppermint Oil

Directions

Shake well and fill dropper with one 10mg serving (30 drops, about 1/2 of dropper). Squeeze drops underneath tongue and hold for 45 seconds before swallowing. Use 1-2 times daily. Store in a cool place out of sunlight.

Typical CBD Nutritional Value Label

Nutrition Facts	
Serving Size 1 dropper (1mL)	
Servings Per Container 15	
Amount Per Serving	
Calories 7	Calories from Fat 7
	% Daily Values*
Total Fat 1g	2%
Saturated Fat 0g	0%
Trans Fat 0g	
Cholesterol 0mg	0%
Sodium 0mg	0%
Total Carbohydrate 0g	0%
Dietary Fiber 0g	0%
Sugars 0g	
Protein 0g	0%

*Percent Daily Values are based on a 2,000 calorie diet. Your Daily Values may be higher or lower depending on your calorie needs.

	Calories	2,000	2,500
Total Fat	Less than	65g	80g
Sat Fat	Less than	20g	25g
Cholesterol	Less than	300mg	300mg
Sodium	Less than	2400mg	2400mg
Total Carbohydrate		300g	375g
Dietary Fiber		25g	30g

An Example of a Price Guide Showing Drops per Container

Taking CBD oil for the first time.

My first CBD purchase was made online and It was a 30ml tincture with 5% CBD and 0.2% THC. I'd never used a tincture before, and I felt a cocktail of emotions before finally trying CBD for the first time. This is what happened.

I loaded up the dropper. CBD oil looks like olive or rapeseed oil with a golden-brown color. Don't spill any onto your clothes or furniture. You'll have a hard time removing the stain since it's mostly oil.

OK I had to start small to see how I reacted to it. I put a couple of drops under my tongue, tried and failed to swish it around my mouth and almost instantly swallowed it. When you first put CBD under your tongue your saliva will quickly appear and make it sometimes tricky to keep the oil in your mouth for a full minute. That's perfectly fine.

It tasted a little earthy and slightly nutty. Not unpleasant and I personally don't see the need to add flavoring to any of the CBD oil I've used. The taste reminded me of the taste of a liquid form of St. Johns Wart which I'd tried years earlier. Most of the taste in CBD oil is coming from the carrier oil which can vary depending on the product. I've seen carrier oil with cloves or sometimes oils are mixed to produce a taste however most unflavored oils taste quite similar.

Although I knew what would happen, I couldn't help expecting to feel instant and noticeable change of some kind. Maybe slightly sleepy or dreamy but no. I didn't feel anything at all initially.

Later that day I took another two small drops and then another before bed. I still felt quite anxious and slightly disappointed that this hadn't really seemed to make my difference so far. I fell asleep a bit quicker than usual and awoke the next day having slept deeply and accompanied with some vivid dreams which still make me chuckle to this day.

So, this was the first little indicator that CBD had done something at least. I took my drops and went about my day. I noticed that I felt ever so slightly groggy for the first half of the morning. Nothing major just a slight heaviness to my eyes which disappeared mod morning and left me feeling fine.

That night I went to the gym as usual and lifted quite heavy weights as part of my routine. Having rested well the night before I felt strong and enjoyed a good quality workout where I pushed myself to lift until failure.

Whenever I do these heavy lifts my heart rate gets elevated as my body recovers from the workout. I always feel it when lying in bed that night however this time it was much less noticeable. This it seemed, was another sign that something had changed.

Over the course of the next few days I was aware that my stress levels were indeed decreased enough for me to notice it. At the same time my concentration levels had slightly increased which had a knock-on effect in my work output along with other areas of my life like writing my books and even playing my guitar.

Sometimes it only takes a small helping hand for your positivity and mental wellbeing to return and for it to become self-propelling. My first experience of CBD did just that and helped be deal with my stress.

Now I know that the mind is a very strange and powerful thing. There's much that we still don't know about how our minds work. Could this uptake in my mood have been brought on by a placebo effect? Could my expectation convince my body that CBD was doing this? It was hard to be sure. I decided to experiment a little.

You know, just to see what happened. I mean, what could possibly go wrong?

Over time I did various tests. Initially it was trying to catch CBD out to see if it was real or not but laterally it was more to test both it and my own boundaries.

It's like when I got my first real high powered sportscar. I was excited and a bit scared and I wanted to know where the cars limits were so that I knew how not to breach them and thus keep me, and it safe. The only way to do this is to push the envelope a little and to see what happens.

Obviously, this search for insight and truths can be dangerous and must be done with the upmost care and respect. I'm never reckless and trust my instincts. I always know when to stop.

Here's some bullet points on my experience so far:

- Mixing 5 or 10% CBD oil with alcohol worked out fine for me with no real adverse effects. Mixing brands or methods of consumptions presented no issues.

- Combining 5 or 10% CBD oil with paracetamol, ibuprofen, co-codamol, antibiotics (amoxicillin) or cough mixtures was fine with no real adverse effects.

- Different brands with the exact same ingredients can still produce slightly different results. Some made me feel sleepy and some didn't. Some made me feel ever so slightly irritable on a moderate dose of 6 drops. The tincture pictured in this book is a 30 ml 5% CBD product from Holland and Barret and this brand makes me feel quite sleepy. It can relax me too however any more than 6 drops and I start feel very slightly irritated. Other brands with the same CBD content and carrier oil seemed to have less effects of any kind.

- Taking CBD on an empty stomach was ok. Effects were still felt within 20 minutes from a tincture.

- CBD didn't help my cold symptoms and it made no real difference to my mood or state of mind when I was sick. It won't help with a chest infection, cough or sore throat.

- It didn't show on a drug test and I never feel fuzzy or tired the next day unless I take the oil later as I've said. Driving or operating machinery isn't a problem for me at all.

- I'm not addicted to CBD. Stopping and starting again is easy and I don't believe that I've built up a tolerance to it. There are no noticeable withdrawal symptoms. There are no visible signs that you take CBD oil and I don't smell or sweat CBD oil smells. I don't need a loading phase with CBD oil like some say. The effects either work quite quickly that same day or don't work at all.

- 5 and 10% Tinctures have worked best for me. I don't mind using the tincture and the natural taste is not an issue for me. I usually take it orally under the tongue or occasionally I put it in food, or I cook with it.

- I took one month's supply of 5% CBD in one evening and suffered no real side effects apart from a dry mouth and a slightly irritated feeling which made my skin feel just a little bit itchy. I also upset stomach the next morning probably due to taking 30ml of oil within a couple of hours. This gave me slight wind although I didn't feel uncomfortable. I slept very soundly that night and the next day I felt a little fuzzy for most of the morning. It cleared, and I felt fine. Overall taking too much CBD didn't cause any lasting harm that I could detect.

- Vapes and sprays didn't work as well as tinctures and capsules for me. Edibles are fine for variety although it can be tricky achieving a precise dosage per serving. CBD isn't cheap and the best value in my opinion comes from the tinctures and concentrates.

- CBD helps my anxiety and insomnia and my wrist pain. The natural feeling of calm helps with other areas like work and even relationships however the effects are not always consistent and sometimes it depends on my state of mind and current fitness levels. It is not always a miracle cure on its own with regards to a health tonic. It certainly lends a helping hand though.

- CBD seems to help balance my partners hormones around period time and it works well with evening primrose. Just a few drops of whatever I'm using at the time helps her.

- CBD works alongside my other healthy habits and occasional supplements including EPA fish oils, macca powder, protein powder, creatine, ZMA tablets and multi vitamins.

- It doesn't make me hungry or suppress my appetite. I don't taste CBD in edibles. The CBD water that I tried didn't taste particularly nice. I'm not a big fan of bottled water though.

- CBD won't cure a hangover unfortunately. And pre-loading with CBD the night before doesn't lessen the chances of or make the ensuing hangover any easier. Milk Thistle is much better in this regard.

- It won't directly affect your sex drive one way or the other. If you take too much oil you might not be bothered doing anything at all apart from sleeping (intense exercise along with lots of seafood or magnesium, zinc and B6 supplements can help your libido)

- It can help me concentrate better and be more productive. It can help me focus during heavy exercise. It helps me with recovery from strength training and it can contribute to a feeling of wellness and positivity.

- Long term use has so far produced no side real effects or problems apart from it being quite expensive for my needs. If my stress levels become severe again, I'll continue to self-medicate as I have done already. I will try to avoid unnatural conventional medications.

- Different products and brands seem to vary slightly in taste and strengths despite showing the same percentage of CBD. Carrier oils used will affect the taste. Some oils darker in color e.g. rapeseed carrier oil is darker than coconut or olive oil. On top of this, people sometimes report that effects were different for them than what others claim. Again, it takes some experimentation to find the right brand that works for you and the sweet spot in the dosage.

- Lotions and salves do work but not as well as tinctures and capsules in my experience.

- CBD makes your skin, hair and nails look a bit healthier. It can generally increase your vitality and energy levels and help towards giving you a healthy glow.

There we are. Overall my experience has been positive so far. No real negatives to report apart from the ambiguous nature of some of the labelling of products and the price of CBD oil. I feel that $80-$100 dollars for a 10% 30ml tincture is quite expensive for a health tonic however if it also removes your chronic pain and helps you sleep then it's money well spent.

My mother is now sleeping better by using the same oil as I use. My Dad however is another matter as he is undertaking a new experimental medication which combines injections and steroids to help with his arthritis. Because much has still to be scientifically tested with CBD, we are reluctant to combine these two treatments at this stage. What he has found so far is that these medications are causing him many unwanted side effects including fatigue and nausea albeit they seem to be helping his arthritis also. We will see how things go from here. He has shown an interest in trying CBD as an alternative in the future.

I visited my Doctor recently and asked if I could have CBD on prescription. I explained that it I'd been self- medicating with it for a long time and that it worked well for me in treating my stress, pain and insomnia. I said that I did not want to go on unnatural medications with unwanted side effects. The conversation went like this.

Dr "Aspirin is natural"

Me "Yes but it has side effects"

Dr "Ah but so does CBD oil!"

Me " Not in my experience it doesn't."

Dr 'Well we couldn't currently justify prescribing CBD as a suitable alternative to conventional medications due to the lack of Scientific data available and due to the budget cuts across the NHS Departments. CBD will most likely become more mainstream and possibly become available on prescription for the issues you mentioned within the next 5-10 years. I see no problem with you continuing to use CBD oil as you have been doing.'

I suspected that the conversation would go along these lines however it was worth asking him anyway. I'm hoping that CBD will be more readily available from the NHS in the future.

Chapter 11: CBD Oil and Your Pets

Not only are you able to use CBD oil to improve your own health, it can also be used to improve the health of your pets. CBD oil is just as effective on your pet as it can be on human beings and there are a ton of great health benefits that come from using it. All mammals can use CBD oil, you just need to make sure that you follow the right dosage (based on size and weight) to ensure that they are able to see the best benefits. Let's look at how CBD oil can be used on your pets and some of the great health benefits they will receive when they start using this product.

What can CBD oil treat in pets?

You might be surprised at how many different things CBD oil is able to do to help your pet. While most pet owners use different medications to help their pets feel better and deal with a variety of common ailments, they can't treat everything. And again, they often come with a lot of harmful side effects. CBD is certainly worth trying, especially if other treatments do not work.

Benefits include:

- Reducing anxiety: Anxiety can be a tough disorder to deal with. Human beings can discuss their feelings and emotions, but your pet is not able to handle anxiety in this way. When the anxiety gets severe enough, it can result in destructive behaviors like scratching, urinating indoors, chewing, and barking. CBD relaxes your pets, so they can stay calm and not react in a negative way. This could be beneficial for animals who are nervous and perhaps made more uncomfortable with loud noises, e.g. roadworks or fireworks.

- Chronic pain relief: When your pet is dealing chronic pain, there are very few options on the market. CBD oil helps keep your pet comfortable because it targets inflammation in the joints. It could also help with dental problems. Not only does it help reduce the amount of pain felt, but it can also help the healing process.

- Loss of appetite: If your pet has trouble eating or has pain and nausea that makes it hard to eat, CBD could do the trick. There are treat options on the market that can provide relief for your pet.

- Seizures: Not only can cannabis help human beings who suffer from seizures, your pet can benefit as well. CBD oil for pets can be used to manage seizures and can reduce their occurrence. This is a huge relief for the pet and for the pet owner, and it will improve your pet's quality of life.

- Aggressive behavior: There are a lot of reasons why your pet may show aggressive behavior. With the help of CBD, you can help calm your pet. It can even help with some stress disorders that your pet experiences, making them healthier and happier.

- IBS: CBD can be used to help treat irritable bowel syndrome in your pet. It has anti-inflammatory properties, so it will make your pet more comfortable. It could help eliminate the disease altogether.

- Glaucoma: Dogs and other animals who are dealing with glaucoma have used CBD. Ingesting CBD sublingually reduces the pressure in the eye. More studies need to be done to see whether this pressure reduction is permanent, but the treatment does provide some temporary relief.

- Heart health: CBD improves cardiac function in dogs suffering from arrhythmia. This can help to reduce the incidences of cardiac events and improves blood flow to most of the major organs.

- Bone health: CBD can also benefit animals that have broken a bone or are dealing with severe osteoporosis. Studies demonstrate how using CBD can stimulate new bone growth while also strengthening bones that are damaged through osteoporosis. Also, there are pain killing and anti-inflammatory properties to CBD which makes it even more ideal.

- Brain: CBD is a powerful neuro-protectant, meaning that it works to protect the nerve cells from issues with impairment, degeneration, and damage. When it is administered after a neurological event or as ongoing treatment for those who have a high likelihood of a neurological event, CBD can help protect the brain from any damage and will reduce the likelihood of a recurrence.

- Diabetes: CBD can help to regulate blood sugar levels and can mitigate the symptoms of diabetes. When it is used correctly, it can reduce damage in the pancreas and, in type 2 diabetes, it can help to improve sensitivity to insulin.

- Immune system: CBD can help with auto-immune illnesses in your pet. It has been effective at regulating the overactive immune system in pets and could reduce the damage that this has on the nature structures and functions of the body.

- Infections: There are several types of bacterial growth that can be slowed down using CBD. Sometimes, it can help to kill bacteria fully. It has been effective in dealing with some medication-resistant bacterial strains.

- Sleep: Dogs with canine cognitive dysfunction were able to enjoy improved sleep patterns by taking CBD oil. This helped them to sleep during the night because it induced drowsiness.

- Psoriasis: While it is rare, your pet could suffer from psoriasis, and CBD can help to treat this disease.

- Muscle relaxant: CBD can help treat not only muscle spasms, but it also works to help with conditions that cause the muscles of your pet to tighten up. It helps them to relax, so that your pet is not so stiff and sore.

- Blood flow: There are numerous reasons that your pet could be suffering from poor blood flow including problems with the valves of their heart and heartworms. The CBD can work to improve circulation and can reduce some of the complications that accompany bad blood flow.

So basically, it can do the same thing for animals as it does for humans. It works with the animals ECS just like it works with ours.

Which pets can use CBD oil?

Almost every animal will be able to benefit from CBD oil. The most common animals to use CBD include cats and dogs, but other mammals can enjoy it as well.

If you are using the CBD on larger animals, it is especially important to talk to your vet before starting this treatment. You will need to give larger doses to these animals because of their size and your vet can make sure you are using it properly and in the right dosage.

What dosage is right for my pet?

Proper dosage is crucial and based on the animal's weight. Initially, it is best to try about 1-5 mg per every 10 pounds of body weight. As always, start with the lowest amount and then increase if needed, just like you would do yourself.

For most cats, you are fine giving them 1mg due to their relatively light weight. For heavier dogs, follow the weight related guidelines. Always monitor how your pet reacts and if there are any major side effects. If there are going to be any changes, these will occur within an hour. If you do not see any changes, then it is time to increase the dosage.

If you are using the CBD for pain relief, the treatment should be given about once every eight hours. If you are using it to correct unwanted behavior in your animal, two times a day is best. Of course, you may need to do more than one treatment to see the improvement you seek.

There is very little risk to overdosing your pet with pure CBD, however if the CBD treatment has trace amounts of THC, make sure to monitor your pet to see any signs of toxicity. Watch them for any signs that they are suffering from a high. This may include your pet having trouble eating, walking, or standing.

CBD can be very helpful to animals. If your pet is dealing with a debilitating ailment, and you want to try a method without harmful side effects, CBD oil may be the answer. Talk to your vet before starting any treatment with your pet. Most vets are familiar with how CBD oil influences animals and they will be able to discuss usage and best practices with you.

CBD Chart for Pets Based on Weight

Pets Weight	Dosage
1 – 20 lbs	1 – 2mg/ 2 - 4 drops
21 – 45 lbs	2 – 3mg/ 4 – 6 drops
46 – 74 lbs	3 – 4mg/ 6 -8 drops
75+ lbs	4 – 5mg/ 8 – 10 drops

Points to remember:

- All animals can benefit from CBD oil. Dosage depends on weight.

- Start with the minimum dose and keep an eye on Rover for signs that he might be high. Reduce dose if required.

- CBD works well in reducing animals' anxiety and calming them down. It has also been very beneficial in reducing inflammation and symptoms of arthritis in animals of all ages.

Chapter 12: Success Stories from Those Who Used CBD Oil

I felt it could be beneficial for you to have a quick look at some cases where CBD has helped people with ailments. There are a lot of people who rely on CBD oil to help them feel better.

Some have been on traditional medications and found that they did not work well. Others wanted to find an all-natural treatment. Here are some of the success stories from CBD oil and from those who were finally able to get some relief by using this product.

- Patient 1: I dealt with chronic headaches that were caused from a traumatic brain injury and a concussion about five years ago. I tried a few other products, and nothing worked. I then decided to try CBD and in just a few weeks, I was pressure and pain free. This was the first time since my accident. In addition, it was also able to help with my mild anxiety that was caused by some hormonal changes after the accident. It also makes it easier for me to focus than ever before.

- Patient 2: I suffer from multiple sclerosis. I have multiple symptoms of MS including insomnia, spasms, fatigue, and headaches. After trying several brands and experimenting with the dosage, I finally found a good nighttime and morning oil to use. Since I started with CBD, I have been able to stop taking my other prescription medications, other than my daily MS medication. Even without these medications, I feel so much better than I have in a long time. And I also have energy I never knew I had!

- Patient 3: I have suffered two strokes in the past four years. After these occurred, I was diagnosed with rheumatoid arthritis. I was often depressed and down in the dumps. I was also lethargic and short-tempered. And the pain I felt from the arthritis meant that it was difficult doing even the smallest tasks. No one wants to live that way. My doctors and specialists gave me lots of drugs, but they never really helped me to feel better. One day, my son called to tell me what he had heard about CBD oil. A few months ago, I decided to start using it. I used one drop, three times a day for a few weeks. Then I increased to two drops of green, two times a day and then two drops of gold at night. I feel a lot better and can enjoy life again.

- Patient 4: For the last 22 years, I have been on disability. I was in so much pain that all I could think about was how to get rid of this pain. As soon as I found the CBD oil, it changed my life. I went down from high pain to mid pain and since I was finally able to get up and move, I started to lose weight. This has helped me to enjoy my life more than ever.

- Patient 5: I suffered from headaches all the time, which usually turned into migraines. My husband fell ill a few years ago, which increased my depression and anxiety. It was hard for me to maintain a happy attitude when I was in so much pain and suffering from depression. Someone from his support group had seen success with CBD oil, so I looked it up and realized it might help me, too. I experimented a bit with the dosage and found taking one drop, three times a day helped to make the headaches go away. It also helped my anxiety diminish and I am slowly weaning off the anti-depressants.

- Patient 6: Two-and-a-half years ago, I was diagnosed with a disease called CVID. I require immunoglobulin infusions for the rest of my life. About nine months after that, I was diagnosed with chronic lymphocytic leukemia. This is all on top of bad migraines for 35 years and fibromyalgia for 25 years. I needed a lot of medications and often felt like I was not functioning well at all. It was at this time I decided to give CBD oil a try. I hoped it would give me some relief from the pain. Within just a few weeks, I got relief from all the pain I had, including migraines, bones, fibromyalgia, and back. After working up to a dose that seemed the best for me, I was able to reduce the pain meds by 75 percent. I still suffer from the diseases, but CBD oil has changed things in a way that allows me to function better.

- Patient 7: CBD has helped me to deal with my fibromyalgia pain. After dealing with this disease for the past 20+ years, it had gotten so bad that I qualified for disability. I spent a lot of time in bed because of the pain, and I suffered from anxiety and depression. I started taking CBD 7 months ago and my body seemed to respond right away. I have less pain and can get more done through the day.

- Patient 8: I have dealt with anxiety for most of my life, and as I've grown older, the panic attacks have worsened. Since I have always been health conscious, I figured that working out and eating right would help take care of it. This did not happen. I decided that 2018 would be the year for me to take care of my mental health, and that is when I came across CBD oil. Since I've started taking it, I have seen a big improvement and have only dealt with one panic attack over the past two months. It has helped me to realize what normal is supposed to feel like.

- Patient 9: I am dealing with severe osteoarthritis, spondylolisthesis, and scoliosis of the spine. All the vertebrae in the back have been fused from T4 down. These fusions were from failed back surgeries, so I have been dealing with chronic pain. CBD oil has helped reduce the pain and allowed me to decrease the use of Norco. I still have some pain, but I feel better and I do not have to worry about being impaired by excessive opioid use.

- Patient 10: I am dealing with an autoimmune disease known as polymyalgia rheumatica. This condition effects the muscles in the hips, shoulders, and neck. I have suffered from chronic inflammation pain for the past ten months and was told that I had to take prednisone to take away the pain. I wanted to find more natural relief. I started taking CBD oil and after just three days, I could feel that my joints were loosening up. Four months later, I still have a bit of discomfort in my shoulders, but I have my life back.

- Patient 11: I suffer from many different diseases. These include anxiety, nausea, migraines, chronic pain, bipolar depression, PTSD, and fibromyalgia pain. My pain was a 10 all day long before I took CBD oil. I never took pain medications because I don't have a tolerance for them, and the few I took for fibromyalgia didn't work and gave a lot of bad side effects. I started using about 350mg of CBD oil for a month. I noticed right away that it helped to calm my anxiety. After one month, I do not feel as nauseous and the pain is less intense. I plan to adjust the dosage to see if it helps even more with some of my disorders.

- Patient 12: Many people in my family have arthritis, fibromyalgia, and lupus. I do as well. The pain got bad last year and made my sleeping problems worse. I couldn't walk after I finished work and did not have any energy to do anything. It was at this time that I heard about CBD oil and I tried it out. I am now able to walk around stores, get to sleep, spend more time with my kids and just live life. And this is after only a week of being on it!

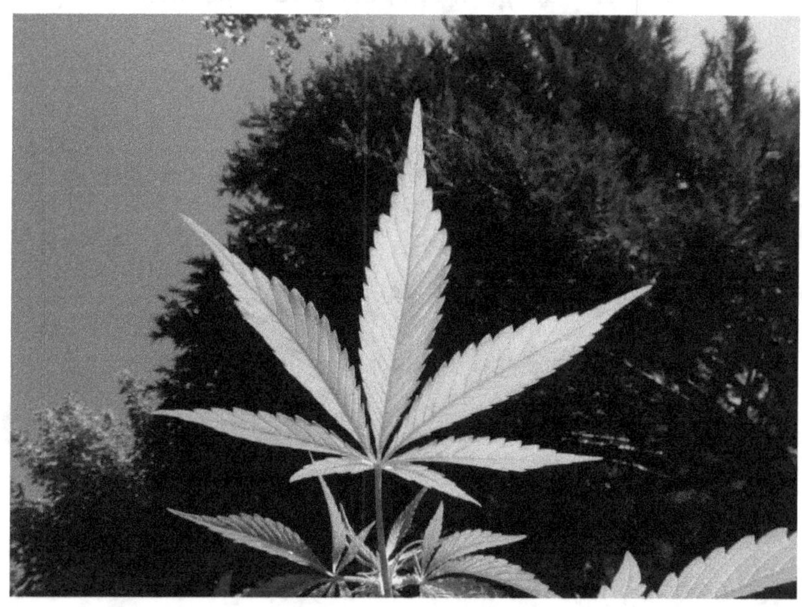

Chapter 11: Cooking with CBD

Cooking with CBD can be a good way of integrating it into your lifestyle especially if you are likely to be taking CBD for a long period of time like me. You can add CBD to just about anything if you avoid exposing it to extreme heat which can kill off the nutrients just like overcooking most foods will potentially destroy most of the nutritional qualities and often the taste as well. Why not have a go at some of these CBD friendly recipes? It's good fun and they are very tasty and easy to make.

Popcorn

Simply add a few drops or squeeze a capsule into your melted butter for some healthy popcorn.

CBD Coconut Oil

Adding cannabidiol to any oil before use gives it a good dose of healthy active compounds.

Drawn Butter

Butter or margarine can easily be given the CBD treatment by just adding a few drops.

CBD-Infused Coffee or Tea

Again add a few drops of tincture or capsule to your favorite brew. Just remember to add it once it's been poured as high heat can kill off the nutrients.

CBD Fruit Smoothies

Blend up yoghurt, banana, raspberries, honey and CBD for a healthy meal supplement or replacement.

Garlic, cream cheese, parmesan cheese and artichoke with a little CBD from a tincture.

Craft Beer

Homebrew or craft brewers work well with CBD. As will wine, spirits, champagne and cocktails.

Chocolate Stout Truffles

12 ounces high-quality dark chocolate chopped

1/2 cup sweetened condensed milk

1/3 cup chocolate stout (or other dark beer)

CBD tincture

pinch salt

cocoa powder and edible gold leaf (optional)

Directions

In a heavy saucepan over low heat, melt chocolate; stir until smooth.

Stir in CBD oil, salt, then liquids a little at a time.

Cool to room temperature.

Shape into one-inch balls; roll in cocoa and top with edible gold leaf.

Store in an airtight container.

Yield: About three dozen

Banana Bread

Ingredients:

1 egg
2 Tbsp. honey
¼ c. cannabis butter
¼ c. buttermilk
1 ½ c. mashed bananas
½ tsp. nutmeg
½ tsp. baking soda
½ tsp. baking powder
½ tsp. salt
¼ c. packed brown sugar
¼ c. sugar
½ c. whole wheat flour
½ c. all-purpose flour
Cooking spray
1 tsp. vanilla

Directions

1. Turn on the oven to 350 degrees. Take out 7 mini-loaf pans and coat them with some cooking spray.
2. Take out a bowl and combine both the flours with the nutmeg, baking soda, baking powder, salt, brown sugar, and sugar.

3. In a second bowl, combine the vanilla, egg, honey, butter, buttermilk, and bananas. Use a mixer to beat these together well.
4. Add the dry ingredients into a bowl and then mix to make combined. Pour this into the loaf pans, just slightly over half full.
5. Add these to the oven and let them bake for 20 minutes, or until the bread is done. Allow them some time to cool on a wire rack for a few minutes before taking out of the pan. Cool a bit longer before serving or storing.

Carrot and Raisin Muffins

Ingredients:

2 tsp. pumpkin pie spice
1 Tbsp. baking powder
1/3 c. packed brown sugar
1 ½ c. all-purpose flour
1 ½ c. raisin bran cereal
2 Tsp. orange zest grated
1 egg
¼ c. vegetable oil
¼ c. cannabis vegetable oil
1 c. carrots shredded
1 c. milk
¾ c. walnuts, chopped
1 c. raisins
½ tsp. salt

Directions:

1. Turn on the oven to 374 degrees. Take out 12 muffin cups and add some paper liners inside.
2. In a bowl, whisk together the orange zest, egg, vegetable oil, cannabis oil, carrots, and milk.
3. In a second bowl, mix together the salt, pumpkin pie spice, baking powder, brown sugar, sugar, flour, and bran flakes.
4. Add the wet ingredients in with the dry ones and then stir to moisten the flour. Stir in the raisins and walnuts.
5. Spoon this into the muffin cups, leaving a little bit of room on the top.
6. Bake these muffins for 25 minutes. Serve them either warm or wait until they have time to cool down first.

Baby Pancakes

Ingredients:
2 Tbsp. confectioners' sugar
Juice from half a lemon
¼ c. butter
1/8 tsp. nutmeg
½ tsp. salt
1 Tbsp. sugar
1 Tbsp. cannabis milk
3 eggs
¾ c. flour
¾ c. milk

Directions

1. Heat up the oven to 425 degrees. Take out a bowl and combine the sugar, cannabis milk, eggs, flour, milk nutmeg, and salt. Stir until there are no lumps.

2. Take out a cast iron skillet and melt the butter over medium heat. When the butter is melted, pour the batter into the pan and then the skillet over to the oven.
3. Bake this mixture for 20 minutes so the pancake has time to become golden brown and puffed.
4. Turn the temperature of the oven down to 300 degrees. Bake this for another 5 minutes before taking the pancake out of the oven.
5. Sprinkle on the sugar and lemon juice before serving.

Mains

Shrimp Creole

Ingredients

1/8 tsp. cayenne pepper
1 bay leaf
1 Tbsp. cannabis oil
2 Tbsp. chopped parsley
1 c. chicken stock
1 can tomatoes, crushed
2 tsp. minced garlic
1 diced celery rib
½ diced green bell pepper
½ diced onion
2 Tbsp. flour
1 Tbsp. olive oil
1 Tbsp. butter
Cooked rice
1 lb. peeled shrimp
Salt

Directions:

1. In a skillet, melt the better and the olive oil. Whisk in the flour and cook until a light roux form. This will take about 4 minutes.
2. Add in the celery, bell pepper, and onion and stir to combine until the vegetables are soft, about 4 minutes.
3. Stir in the garlic and cook for another minute. After that time, stir in the tomatoes with their juices, the salt, cayenne, bay leaf, cannabis oil, parsley, and stock.
4. Increase the heat to bring this to a boil and then reduce to a simmer to cook for 15 minutes.
5. Add in the shrimp, stirring to combine, and cook another 5 minutes until the shrimp is done. Remove the bay leaf and serve over rice.

Honey Lime Chicken

Ingredients:
2 c. cooked rice
Scallions
2 tsp. toasted sesame seeds
½ tsp. sesame oil
1 tsp. ginger
1 tsp. sriracha hot sauce
2 Tbsp. lime juice
2 Tbsp. cannabis honey
6 Tbsp. honey
½ c. light soy sauce
Pepper
Salt
1 chicken sliced into 8 pieces

Directions:

1. Turn on the grill to 375 degrees. Use the pepper and salt to season the chicken pieces. Cook on the grill until cooked through.
2. While your chicken cooks, prepare the glaze. Take out a pan and combine the rest of the ingredients, except the rice.
3. Heat over the stove, stirring until it starts to bubble. Reduce the heat and cook until it is thick, another three minutes.
4. Place the chicken into a bowl and toss to coat with the glass. Garnish and serve over rice.

Snacks and Desserts

Caramel Corn

Ingredients:

1 tsp. vanilla
¾ tsp. baking soda
2 tsp. salt
¼ c. honey
1 c. dark brown sugar
1 Tbsp. cannabis butter
1/3 c. butter
12 c. popped popcorn, plain

Directions;

1. Preheat the oven to 225 degrees. Take out two baking sheets and line with parchment paper.
2. Place your popcorn in a bowl. Bring out a pan and melt the cannabis butter and butter. Stir in with the salt, honey,

and brown sugar. Stir this on the stove until the mixture starts to boil.

3. Lower the heat to a simmer. Cook for about 90 seconds. Take the pan from the heat and add in the vanilla and baking soda. Pour over the popcorn and toss to coat before it hardens.

4. Spread this onto the baking sheets and put into the oven. Bake for 15 minutes.

5. Take out of the oven currently and stir around the popcorn to break up the pieces. Allow to cook for another 15 minutes.

Chocolate Chip Cookies

Ingredients:
1 c. chocolate chips
½ tsp. salt
½ tsp. baking soda
1 1/8 c. flour
1 egg
1 tsp. vanilla
¼ c. butter
¼ c. cannabis butter
2/3 c. brown sugar
2/3 c. sugar

Directions:

1. Turn the oven on to 375 degrees. While that is heating up, bring out a bowl and beat the vanilla, butter, cannabis butter, brown sugar, and sugar together until creamy. Beat in the egg next.

2. In a second bowl, stir together the salt, baking soda, and flour. When those are combined, beat them into the butter mixture along with the chocolate chips.
3. Drop some of the cookie dough onto baking sheets and then place into the oven to bake.
4. After 15 minutes, take the cookies out of the oven and serve warm.

Brownies

Ingredients:

¾ c. macadamia nuts
½ tsp. vanilla
3 eggs
1 c. brown sugar
4 ½ oz. chocolate
¼ c. cannabis coconut oil
1/3 c. coconut oil
¾ tsp. salt
2 Tbsp. cocoa powder
¾ c. flour

Directions:

1. Turn on the oven to 350 degrees. Bring out a bowl and combine the salt, cocoa powder, and flour.
2. In a pan, melt the chocolate, cannabis coconut oil, and coconut oil together over a low heat. When these are melted, set aside and let cool for five minutes.
3. After that time, stir in the brown sugar along with the vanilla and the egg. Add in the flour mixture and the nuts.

4. When this is ready, pour onto some prepared baking pans and put into the oven. Bake for 30 minutes until they are done. Take out of the oven and allow to cool before serving.

Beauty Products with CBD Oil

Body Lotion

Ingredients:

.5-gram CBD isolate
2 c. olive oil
Favorite essential oil (4 drops)

Directions:

1. Mix the three ingredients together so that the CBD isolate can dissolve and get mixed into the solution.
2. Use this on any part of the body that needs some body lotion or that is experiencing pain.
3. If you add in some salt and a little lavender oil, you can make a good body scrub with the oil.

Easy Salve

Ingredients:

1 oz. shea butter
1 oz. beeswax
1 c. CBD infused oil

Directions:

1. Create a double boiler by adding a smaller pot on top of a larger pot with a few inches of water in the bottom.
2. Add in the oil and the beeswax after the oil is at a gentle simmer. Make sure to stir this around often.
3. When the beeswax is almost dissolved, add in the shea butter. Continue to stir until it dissolves completely.
4. Pour this into your chosen containers. Let them set for a few hours to become completely solid.
5. Use when needed.

Anti-Wrinkle Cream

Ingredients:

1 Tbsp. confectioner's cream
1 tsp. vanilla
1 c. cream, heavy
7 g. CBD oil

Directions:

1. Add the oil and the cream to a double boiler. Let the heat be low and simmer these for an hour.
2. After that time, let the cream cool down a bit and then put into a container in the fridge to make cold.
3. Chill your whisk and a large bowl in a freezer for about ten minutes.
4. Take them from the freezer and then add in the prepared cream to it. Whip with a whisk to make some stiff peaks.

Beat in the vanilla and sugar until peaks form. Use this on your skin, rubbing in gently to get the best results.

Appendix: Common Terms to Know

Here is a quick reference to help you understand if you get stuck during reading or if you just need a reminder:

- Agricultural hemp: The varieties of *Cannabis Sativa L.* The plant contains less than 0.3 percent of THC in the dry weight, and it is grown mostly for industrial purposes. This product is legal for use in the United States and more than 40 other countries.

- *Cannabis Sativa L.*: A species of plant that is found in the genus *Cannabis*. It will refer to both marijuana and agricultural hemp, two completely different plants that are both sub species of cannabis.

- CBD: Short for cannabidiol, a Phyto cannabinoid that is found in cannabis. It is the part that can provide a lot of health benefits to animals and humans.

- Endocannabinoid: Naturally occurring cannabinoids found in the human body. When these do not work properly or there are not enough, it can take the body out of balance and make you feel unwell.

- Endocannabinoid system: The system of endocannabinoids and the enzymes that are responsible for regulating the production of endocannabinoids, and their receptors all together

- CB1: A cannabinoid receptor that is found mostly in the central nervous system. This includes the nerves of the spinal cord and the brain.

- CB2: Another type of cannabinoid receptor found mostly in the peripheral nervous system, the nerves that control the body outside of the spinal cord and brain.

- THC: Short for tetrahydrocannabinol. THC is a Phyto cannabinoid found in cannabis and can have some health benefits of animals and humans. However, this chemical is responsible for intoxicating effects that are common with marijuana use, so some people are not fond of using it.

- Entourage effect: The idea that biologically active compounds may have more biological activity when you administer them with other inactive compounds, rather than on their own.

- Hemptourage effect: The entourage effect of the compounds that are found inside of hemp-derived CBD oil and help optimize your wellness and health.

- CO2 extraction: A method used to extract the CBD from the plant. Pressurized CO2 gas (safe, liquid form) is used to extract the oil from the plant. It has the advantage of not having a residue with the final product.

- Non-psychotic: The substance or chemical has no effects on the behavior, personality, or the mind of the user. The user does not get high.

- Hemostasis: The self-regulating process where the body tries to find its balance.

Conclusion

CBD is a hot topic and it has been thrust into the limelight recently with some high-profile cases which clearly show that CBD oil has significant health benefits that simply cannot be ignored.

This has forced Government departments to have a closer look at the antiquated laws that currently surround CBD products. There has also been a definite shift in public sentiment towards CBD and I believe that this will be the catalyst that starts the chain of events which will bring about a major Worldwide change in the current laws.

It's started happening already and attitudes to cannabis are slowly changing. As this change gathers more momentum it will attract the attention of the big pharmaceutical companies who will be keen show us scientific proof that this new CBD product they're selling has fact based and proven benefits.

We're already starting to see celebrity endorsements of CBD products and loads of new advertisements selling CBD products. Interestingly the tone of these adverts is wholesome, healthy and organic. In ways this logical progression is a good thing because the current lack of scientific based evidence is making some people question the validity of the health claims of CBD oil.

The public needs to be educated and given the solid facts so that they can make an informed decision on whether to try CBD oil for themselves and disperse the myths and untruths that are tied to cannabis in general.

The UK has relaxed its stance a little and will allow the use of Medical Marijuana to patients suffering from the effects of epilepsy, chemotherapy and MS only once every other drug has been tried and shown not to work. There are over 10 million people suffering from chronic pain un the UK alone and only one pharmaceutical company who is licensed to produce and distribute Medical Marijuana.

People who cannot get a doctor to prescribe them what they know will work for them will simply continue to do what they've always done and go straight to the black market which, according to the Government, will in turn fuel organized criminal activity.

The Government could take control of this trade just like it has done in the past with alcohol and tobacco, and generate billions in revenue which could help create financial equality in our society, or build more homes or hospitals or they could use this money for more research into cancer or dementia or any number of other good causes. They could even wipe out the so-called financial deficit which none of us caused but are paying for regardless.

Now of course each one of us is different. CBD will almost certainly help most people but not everyone. The best way to find out if CBD will work for you is for you to take the information in this book and then try the oil for yourself. Just be bold and give it a go. What have you got to lose? It might change your life. If you experiment with the different brands in this book the chances are that you will find one that does something for you and then it will be up to you to decide on how you want to use the oil in your life.

There are many online groups and forums where you can connect with other CBD users and share your experiences. These places offer a wealth of information and you don't need to post if you don't want to but asking specific questions can be a very good way of gaining more knowledge. Why not have a look on

Facebook and twitter for CBD Hemp groups and join them. I am part of several of these groups and I can tell you that they are very interesting and useful for beginners and experienced CBD users. It's very easy to join and some of these groups even run reviews and testimonials of various CBD products and offer discounts. Why not give it a go? You have nothing to lose and everything to gain.

You made it until the end!

Thank you for taking the time to read this book. If you have enjoyed the read, then please nip on to amazon and leave an honest review.
It will also really help other people decide if the book will help them.

Thank you and I wish you the very best of luck!

Here's a final thought:

You can be the person you deserve to be.
You have the power to change your life.
You don't need to settle for anything less.
Start right now!

Les Brown